More Praise for

THE PLAGUE CYCLE

"This year's must-read . . . If you want to understand the current Covid-19 crisis and be prepared for what is likely to come next, read this book."

—Richard Florida, author of *The Rise of the Creative Class*

"[This] would be fascinating at *any* time, but during the current pandemic it provides a critical historical and analytic perspective for policymakers, scholars, and interested laypeople thinking about how to address Covid-19."

—Michael Kremer, professor at Harvard University and winner of the Nobel Prize in Economics

"Lively writing . . . Kenny peppers the broad sweep of his [history] with vivid examples."

—Financial Times

"An absorbing history . . . I hope everyone will read this and do all they can to get across the message of eternal vigilance in this 'unending war.'"

—Diane Coyle, Bennett Professor of Public Policy at the University of Cambridge

"Full of historical nuggets . . . The most important parts of the book are undoubtedly those that say something larger about human behavior."

—*The Sunday Times* (UK)

"An astute explication of our species' battles with microbes since the dawn of human time. An optimist, Kenny argues that humanity has the tools to conquer infectious diseases."

—Laurie Garrett, author of *The Coming Plague*

"Infectious disease has always been with us and arguably always will be. Charles Kenny's book is a lively survey of our millennia-long struggle to defeat it."

—*Daily Mail* (UK)

"Throughout history, infectious diseases have been defeated. Covid-19 will be defeated too. Charles Kenny's brilliant *The Plague Cycle* is the book of the hour."

—Gregg Easterbrook, author of *It's Better Than It Looks*

"A very easy read. Kenny has a light touch even when explaining the most serious and complicated of arguments."

—*The Diplomat*

"Compelling . . . Kenny reminds us that nothing unites us, or divides us, as powerfully as our infectious diseases."

—Kyle Harper, author of *The Fate of Rome: Climate, Disease, and the End of an Empire*

"A timely, lucid look at the role of pandemics in history."

—*Kirkus Reviews*

"A concise, erudite, and highly readable narrative probing humanity's protracted and Malthusian battle against deadly pathogens."

—**Timothy C. Winegard, author of *The Mosquito: A Human History of Our Deadliest Predator***

"In his fact-filled and alarming overview of major infectious diseases past and present, economist Kenny discusses sources and vectors of epidemics, the toll of suffering and death, progress in controlling communicable diseases, and persistent problems."

—***Booklist* (starred review)**

"Important, timely, and also gripping . . . Fit to stand beside William H. McNeill's *Plagues and Peoples.*"

—**David Wootton, author of *Bad Medicine: Doctors Doing Harm Since Hippocrates* and *The Invention of Science***

"Kenny contextualizes the Covid-19 pandemic. . . . A worthy primer on a subject of pressing importance."

—***Publishers Weekly***

"Well written, sweeping . . . An excellent treatment on the history of infectious diseases and the complex relationship with human societies."

—**Byron Carson, American Institute for Economic Research**

"Accessible . . . Informative and colorful history."

—***Library Journal***

“Splendid . . . The intellectual strength of *The Plague Cycle* is its use of thorough historical analysis. . . . Truly, this is tip-top!”

—**Dorothy Porter, author of *Health, Civilization and the State***

“[A] gem.”

—***The Independent* (Ireland)**

THE PLAGUE CYCLE

The Unending War Between Humanity and Infectious Disease

CHARLES KENNY

SCRIBNER

New York London Toronto Sydney New Delhi

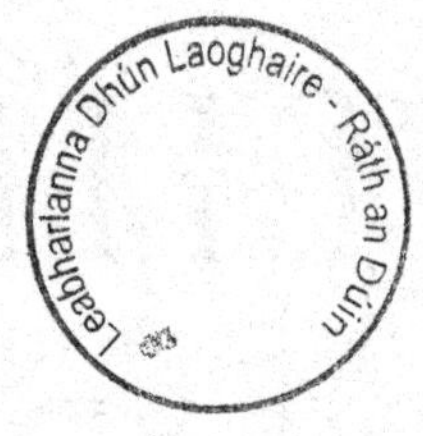

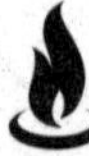

Scribner
An Imprint of Simon & Schuster, Inc.
1230 Avenue of the Americas
New York, NY 10020

First Scribner trade paperback edition October 2021

SCRIBNER and design are registered trademarks of The Gale Group, Inc., used under license by Simon & Schuster, Inc., the publisher of this work.

For information about special discounts for bulk purchases, please contact Simon & Schuster Special Sales at 1-866-506-1949 or business@simonandschuster.com.

The Simon & Schuster Speakers Bureau can bring authors to your live event. For more information or to book an event, contact the Simon & Schuster Speakers Bureau at 1-866-248-3049 or visit our website at www.simonspeakers.com.

Manufactured in the United States of America

1 3 5 7 9 10 8 6 4 2

Library of Congress Cataloging-in-Publication Data has been applied for.

ISBN 978-1-9821-6533-8
ISBN 978-1-9821-6534-5 (pbk)
ISBN 978-1-9821-6535-2 (ebook)

Contents

Preface

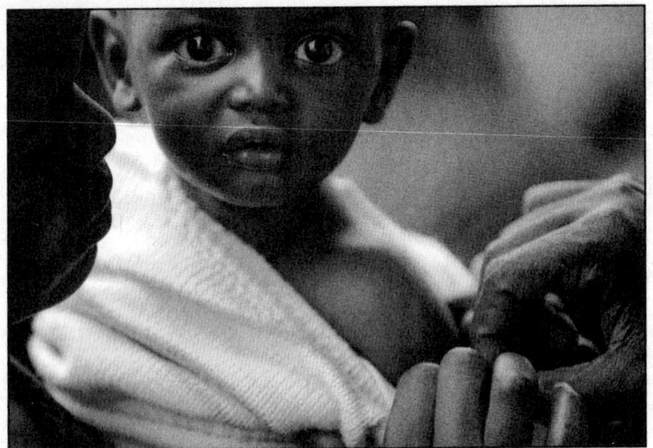

A child isn't too sure about being vaccinated against measles. (Credit: "Not Sure About the Vaccination" by Julian Harneis is licensed under [CC BY-SA 2.0])

The two leading killers worldwide at the start of the twenty-first century are heart attacks and strokes. That is evidence of humanity's greatest triumph: until recent decades, most people didn't live long enough to die of heart failure. Rather, they were felled by a range of infectious diseases that picked off the young or swept through whole populations in pandemic catastrophe.

Covid-19 is a terrible reminder that our victory against infection is far from complete—and in all likelihood *never* will be complete. The cycle of population growth, pandemic, and recovery isn't nearly as violent as it has been in the past, but it's still with us. Many more infectious diseases have emerged over the past century than have been eradicated. And the coronavirus has demonstrated the immense costs we bear when people are forced to rely on one of the very earliest responses to infection: running from it.

But although 2020 marked a tragic global reversal, recent progress against infection has been remarkable. In 2015, as I started to think about writing this book, I crowded into a small basement room of the Seattle Westin Hotel with hundreds of doctors, public health workers, and researchers for an event called "Lessons Learned on the Path to Eradication." The humbleness of the setting aside, the people who were onstage should be world famous for the contributions they've made: Jeffrey Mariner, of Tufts University, created a stable vaccine against the cattle disease rinderpest. Pedro Alonso directed the Global Malaria Program at the World Health Organization. Frank Richards, from the Carter Center, battled diseases caused by parasitic worms. Chris Elias, at the Gates Foundation, led his organization's polio eradication effort. And Bill Foege developed the global smallpox eradication strategy rolled out by the World Health Organization in the 1970s.

Of the infectious killers these five speakers worked to stamp out, two have already been driven to extinction, two are on the verge of eradication, and as for the remaining scourge, wiping it out is a real possibility within our lifetimes. In 1980, the smallpox eradication campaign succeeded. Hundreds of millions died of smallpox in the first eight decades of the twentieth century. But since then only one person, a lab technician, has died of the disease—infected from an accidental release of a scientific sample. Rinderpest was wiped out globally in 2011, ending a disease that killed millions of cattle owned by some of the planet's very poorest households. Rinderpest was also the likely source of the human mass murderer measles. Unchecked, it could have mutated into a species-hopping version once again. The number of cases of guinea worm (a parasite that causes excruciating blisters, vomiting, and dizziness) has fallen by more than 99.9 percent worldwide over the past two decades. As of April 2020, the wild polio virus (which can cripple and kill) had been limited to two countries. And since 2000, thirty-four countries worldwide, including China, Argentina, and South Africa, have made massive strides toward eliminating malaria, cutting death rates by an average of 87 percent.[1]

These and earlier victories have been won through the combined efforts of billions of people. Among them are Lady Mary Wortley Montagu, who popularized variolation—the first effective protection against smallpox; Edward Jenner, who experimented with cowpox to create the first vaccine; Ali Maow Maalin, the last person to contract smallpox outside the laboratory, who spent the rest of his life fighting polio; and Salma Farooqi, who was tortured and killed by the Taliban for the crime of vaccinating children against that same disease.

I would argue that these people are heroes in a worldwide struggle for better health that has seen massive progress in recent decades, but "hero" and "progress" are both controversial words in a book that discusses history. The concern is perhaps best illustrated by a review of David Wootton's 2006 book *Bad Medicine: Doctors Doing Harm Since Hippocrates*. Wootton is a historian at the University of York and his *Bad Medicine* argues that doctors before the twentieth century did little if anything to improve health outcomes of their patients. Wootton offers explanations as to why that was the case. The book's reviewer, Harvard historian Steven Shapin, claimed *Bad Medicine* wasn't history because it documented and celebrated progress, naming heroes. The job of the historian of science, Shapin argued, isn't to judge but to interpret and understand the past in its own terms.

Wootton countered that since both he and Shapin agreed there'd been genuine and substantial medical progress, there was nothing wrong in writing a narrative of that progress.[2] I agree with Wootton, even if that might alienate some historians.[3]

And there *is* something to appreciate in the fact that average life expectancy at birth worldwide has climbed from below thirty in the 1870s to above seventy today. Such innovations as sewer systems, sterilization, vaccination, and use of antibiotics are important reasons why.

In the months I was completing this book, a lot of my thinking and writing was about Covid-19 and possible ways to limit its devastating effect on our health and the economy. The pandemic has elevated a whole new set of heroes in the fight against infectious disease, from nurses and doctors to shelf stockers and delivery staff. Thanks to people like them, I know we'll continue striking blows against premature death.

CHAPTER ONE

Malthus's Ultimate Weapon

> Premature death must in some shape or other visit the human race.
>
> —Malthus

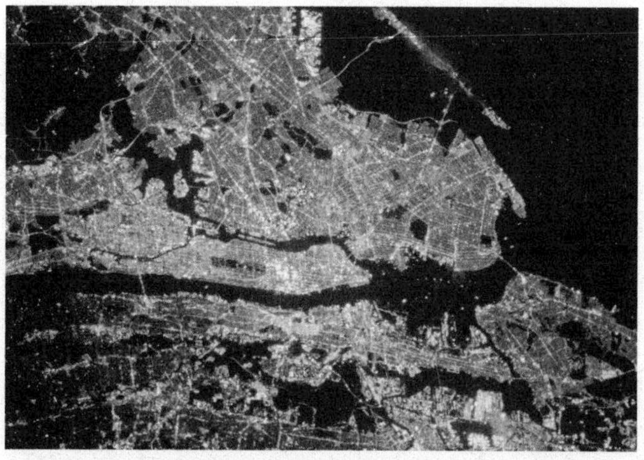

New York today has a population twice as large as the entire world in 10,000 BCE. That is only possible because of victories over infection. (Credit: NASA)

To understand the scale of the health revolution of the last 150 years, we must grasp the magnitude of the trap humanity escaped. It was a trap laid out elegantly (if somewhat inaccurately) by Thomas Robert Malthus in his book *An Essay on the Principle of Population.*

Robert was the seventh child in his family. He went to Cambridge University and excelled, becoming a fellow at Jesus College. He also joined the Church of England, and it was while he was a curate in Surrey that he wrote his *Essay*, first published in 1798 during the early stages of Britain's Industrial Revolution.

The book presented a grim law of population: given humanity's capacity to breed, unchecked populations would rapidly expand. As populations multiplied, more people would use the same land for hunting or farming, or begin to work lower-quality land. This would reduce overall output per person—and the amount that each could consume would decline in lockstep. The number of people would continue to increase until their consumption was reduced to a minimum.

If populations continued to rise beyond that, people wouldn't have enough to eat. That in turn would increase mortality—from disease, famine, or violence. In the end, thanks to a rising death rate, populations would shrink, and output per person remaining would rise. That would bring consumption back to its subsistence level. Scientific progress wouldn't help escape this vicious cycle: marginal improvements in efficiency and output thanks to technology advances like better tools for hunting, heavier plows, or new seeds would simply be eaten up by the hungry mouths of an expanded population. In short, humanity might rise or fall in absolute numbers, but the bulk of the populace would forever live brutish lives on the edge of subsistence.

Malthus's theory couldn't have been more pessimistic. Historically, he maintained, there were only three ways to check population growth: vice, misery, or restraint. For the eighteenth-century parson, vices included prostitution, venereal disease, homosexuality, and birth control.

Misery, the usual alternative to vice, included war, pestilence, and famine. Malthus waxed poetic on this subject:

> The power of population is so superior to the power of the earth to produce subsistence for man, that premature death must in some shape or other visit the human race. The vices of mankind are active and able ministers of depopulation. They are the precursors in the great army of destruction, and often finish the dreadful work themselves. But should they fail in this war of extermination, sickly seasons, epidemics, pestilence, and plague advance in terrific array, and sweep off their thousands and tens of thousands. Should success be still incomplete, gigantic inevitable famine stalks in the rear, and with one mighty blow levels the population with the food of the world.[1]

To avoid vice and misery acting as grim checks to population, the only course was restraint: Malthus's forlorn hope was that moral purity could help most of humanity raise itself above a life of bare subsistence. To keep populations low meant marrying virginal, late, and frigid. Minimal indulgence in sex would produce very few babies, which would help ensure higher living standards and longer lives for the children that *were* born. Malthus himself married at thirty-eight, and had only two children. But he had little confidence that the mass of people would follow his lead.

Pessimistic Malthus may have been, but in the years that preceded his analysis, his theory broadly lined up with the facts: populations rose or declined as circumstances changed, but the average person planet-wide consumed so little that they lived considerably below the poverty line of today's poorest nations. And all three methods outlined by Malthus have played their role in limiting population. In some cases, humans have lowered birth rates—sometimes by methods the good reverend would consider virtuous, often by those he'd consider vice-ridden. In most cases, the misery of war, pestilence, and famine have played the larger part.

In prehistory, infectious disease was widespread enough to play a large role in human evolution. But it still played a comparatively minor role in death, particularly when humans began to migrate out of Africa, outrunning many of the infections of their birthplace.[2] What caused infectious disease to begin regaining the upper hand was when farming became a substitute source of sustenance. As it turned out, large-scale infection was the poxed handmaiden of agriculture and civilization. As humanity packed together with animals in crowded cities and villages, for example, influenza jumped from pigs (or possibly ducks) to infect humans. And other microbes leveraged proximity to do their own spreading.

For most of the time civilization has existed, pestilence has wiped out far more lives than famine and violence combined—so much so that Malthus's proposed final limit of land and resources as the check to human numbers has rarely been approached. Disease has usually kept populations below the levels that could have been supported given agricultural technologies at the time. In Malthus's language, famine did indeed "stalk in the rear"—not least because infectious diseases become bigger killers as more people share the same space. They're a self-regulating tool of population control. The expansion of civilization—and, in particular, of cities—was limited by the very diseases it had enabled.

The rise and spread of civilizations, and the growing trade between them, provided parasites with unprecedented reach. As empires rose in Europe and China, and were linked by trade across the Asian steppe, new populations were exposed to diseases. Plague twice brought low much of Eurasia. The first time that occurred, it helped doom the Roman Empire and enabled the rise of Islam in its southern territories. Plague struck again toward the second half of the fourteenth century, when the Black Death wiped out a significant percentage of humanity.

When Europeans discovered the New World, so did their pathogens. Great empires in the Americas were shattered thanks in considerable part to the onslaught of Old World diseases that arrived with Columbus or those who followed him. When Africans were brought in to replace native populations as slaves, they carried with them some of humanity's oldest infections, including deadlier strains of malaria. The indigenous population of the New World fell to less than one-tenth of its level of 1491 as a result. More than three hundred years after Columbus, Malthus still wrote of the Americas as a place of small populations with an abundance of land. Meanwhile, by removing vast numbers through the violence of slavery and the introduction of new infections by expanding slave trade networks, Europeans also reduced Africa's population.

But if globalization was a vehicle for the launch of pandemics, it's also true that it was severely limited by the very same diseases:

empire building constantly faltered thanks to plague and tropical fevers. Conquest, colonization, and trade were all severely curtailed by the death rates faced by imperial adventurers in alien disease environments.

By the time of the last great die-offs of populations previously unexposed to Eurasian disease, the world was on the verge of dramatic progress against infection. At the beginning of the nineteenth century, it was still fair to argue that living standards for England's poorest were little higher than in any previous point in history, and their health possibly worse. The most effective and widespread response to infection remained avoidance—flight, quarantine, and access restrictions. But as the century progressed, Britain (followed by Europe and North America) saw rising population and living standards and, at the same time, falling mortality. Thanks to a revolution in sanitation, infection was on the retreat. And due to a combination of techniques, including some Malthus would have considered unconscionable, birth rates began to fall, too. It was an irony that the Malthusian model started to break down completely just as Malthus was writing his *Essay*.

In the twentieth century, with a medical revolution that included vaccination and antibiotics, progress against premature death spread worldwide. From the vicious Malthusian cycle of better health guaranteeing poverty, the medical revolution helped create a virtuous cycle of health and productivity reinforcing each other. Everywhere, the reverend's miseries seemed to be in retreat. Famine, pestilence, and war all reduced their toll in the second half of the century, but the number of people saved by reduced infection was by far the largest.

Global efforts against infection over the past two centuries—from washing hands to constructing sewer systems to making use of penicillin, immunization, and bed nets—have saved billions from premature death and billions more from stunted growth, pain, paralysis, blindness, or a lifetime of recurring fever. Two hundred years ago, almost half of all people born died before their fifth birthday, mostly from infection. Today, that figure is below *one in twenty-five.*[3] And we've passed a huge milestone in the last few years—more people worldwide are dying from noninfectious diseases than from infectious ones. For all the suffering and deaths they've caused, new pandemics, including Covid-19, haven't reversed that trend.

The changes wrought by the decline of infectious death have been as seismic as its rise—affecting everything from global power to the nature of home life. Not least, lowered infection risk unleashed urbanization and globalization. Sanitation and the medical revolution have allowed these processes to explode so that ever more of the world's population lives in globally connected cities.

But the effects of victories against infection have gone far beyond bringing people together. They're a major factor in declining birth rates, because it turns out child survival is a great preventative when it comes to having further children. From a historical average of six children or more, the average woman worldwide now has between two and three.[4] That has led to the global emergence of the nuclear family and the aging of populations. Lower infection and its impacts are also factors behind the explosion in global education (because parents who have fewer children can afford to invest more in those they do have), the emancipation of women (since they're freed from endless child-rearing), and economic dynamism (because healthy and educated populations are more productive). The end result is a world with a far healthier population some seven times larger than in Reverend Malthus's day, living on an average income four times greater than that of world-leading Britain in 1775.[5]

Millions still die every year of easily prevented or cured conditions, but the Malthusian trap has been sprung. The question remains as to whether it will stay open. How the fight against infection progresses will help shape the future of global civilization: how many people will live on the planet, how sustainably, and even how peacefully. If victories against infection have allowed us to get closer, to live with millions and travel worldwide, the coronavirus lockdowns and social distancing are a painful illustration of the psychological, social, and economic costs when we're pushed apart again by a renewed threat of disease.

That's the irony of our progress against death from infection over the past two centuries. It has helped create the perfect environment for the emergence of a new disease outbreak and the perfect environment for that outbreak to have catastrophic social and economic impact. The world's population (human and livestock alike) has never been as large, nor commerce so global, nor peace so widespread. Covid-19 is only the latest in a succession of new infections that have emerged and spread in our closer and connected world. Before the current novel coronavirus were previous coronaviruses—as well as AIDS, Ebola, and bird flu.

At the same time, we're abusing our most effective tools against disease—misusing antibiotics by feeding them to farm animals in bulk; leaving our children unvaccinated; funding research on new bioweapons while underfunding new vaccines, treatments, and cures; and letting weak medical systems fester in the world's poorest countries. And our reaction to disease too often echoes that of our distant forebears; at a time when global human interaction is central to our wealth and welfare, we call for flight bans and trade restrictions. Globally, we respond to new infectious threats too late. We don't prepare and we don't coordinate.

We have to do better for next time, because there *will* be a next time. Phenomena ranging from evolution to climate to demographics mean that many infectious diseases tend to follow cycles: flu seasons move back and forth between hemispheres in a regular yearly pattern. Epidemics of diseases like measles and smallpox would strike every few years or decades as the number of new potential victims in a community climbed. The plague of the Black Death spread mass mortality in the sixth, the fourteenth, and the late nineteenth century at times of instability combined with closer global connections. And some epidemiologists argue that we're in the midst of a new stage of an even longer cycle. After a *first* transition toward greater disease threats sparked by the rise of farming, followed by a *second* transition toward reduced threat thanks to interventions including sanitation, vaccines, and antibiotics, we're now in a *third* epidemiological transition back toward greater infectious risk as a result of emerging new diseases spread worldwide by globalization.

This last idea likely underestimates humanity's ability to respond to disease threats. We are flattening the plague cycle. But through sufficient neglect or miscalculation, we could allow communicable diseases to fight back and reclaim their place as death's most popular weapon. History suggests such a reversal would shape the coming century more than almost any other conceivable event—more than climate change, far closer to limited thermonuclear war. And even if that full threat doesn't materialize, we could allow poor response to new diseases like Covid-19 to stifle global progress.

But at least recent history suggests humanity's response to the new threat *can* be rapid and effective if we so choose. And that reassures us that humanity in the twenty-first century is in a considerably better position in the fight against infection than earlier generations. Because for most of humanity's time on the planet, effective responses never came.

CHAPTER TWO

Civilization and the Rise of Infection

Being subject therefore to so few causes of sickness, man, in the state of nature, can have no need of remedies.

—Rousseau

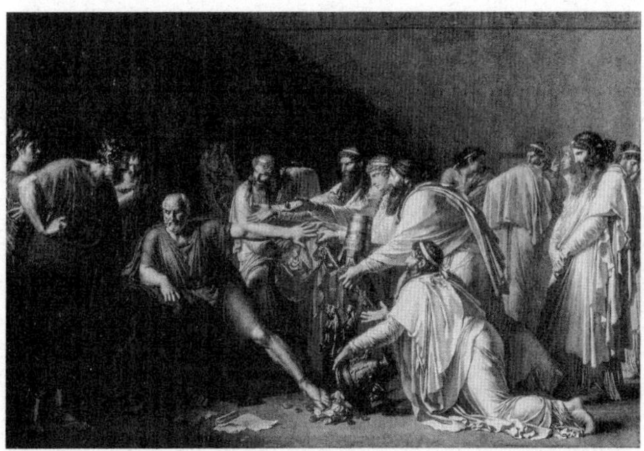

Hippocrates, the "father of medicine" who'd treated victims in the plague of Athens, refuses gifts from the Persian king Artaxerxes, who is seeking the same help in dealing with a plague in his country. (Source: *Hippocrates Refusing the Gifts of Artaxerxes.* A. L. Girodet-Trioson, 1792. Wikimedia Commons)

"Mitochondrial Eve," as she was called, was a creation of scientific theory based on genetic analysis of her offspring—namely, us. In 1987, a team of population geneticists analyzed mitochondrial DNA from 147 people around the world. This segment of genetic code at the heart of every one of our cells is passed down from mothers—and only mothers—to sons and daughters. Using estimates of how long it takes DNA to mutate, the researchers calculated the time needed for all of the existing mitochondrial material around in humans today to have evolved from a single ancestral source. That single source they labeled Mitochondrial Eve. In theory, everyone on the planet today is her direct descendant, and she's the most recent human of which that can be said.

According to the DNA evidence, our common ancestor was alive more than one hundred thousand years ago.[1] Mitochondrial Eve would have lived with a small tribe of people. Hunting and gathering takes a lot of land per person for food, so large communities simply aren't practical.[2] She lived far before the dawn of civilization and the rise of agriculture and cities. And she lived before the time when many of the world's greatest infectious killers had evolved and spread—diseases including smallpox, measles, and the flu.

Even so, there were many prehistoric parasites afflicting mankind. One example may have been the guinea worm, now near the edge of eradication. Larvae of the worm float in pools of water until a lucky few are swallowed by the cyclops—a small water flea. Once inside they grow, feast on the flea's ovaries or testes, and wait for their host to get swallowed in turn—by a human drinking the water. This isn't pleasant for the flea—or for us. As the cyclops dissolves in human digestive juices, the more robust guinea worm larva burrows through the human's intestine and settles briefly in the abdominal wall. If the female larva finds a male to impregnate her, she eventually makes her way to the leg, where she hooks on, feeds, and grows over the course of a year—up to a yard in length. Most of that distance is made up by a hugely distended uterus packed with half a million embryos.

The human host suffers from an irritating blister at the end of the worm. When it bursts, the wound reveals the uterus. To relieve the burning and itching, the victim often stumbles to the nearest water hole to douse the blister. As he or she does, the worm ejects embryos, releasing the next generation of guinea worms back into the pool.[3] Clinical parasitologist Rosemary Drisdelle argues that the worm might be the origin of the fiery serpent that wraps around the rod of Asclepius as the symbol of medicine—because the traditional way of removing the guinea worm is to wrap its end around a stick and slowly, over the course of a month, wind the body around it until the whole worm is pulled out.

Confronting, hunting, and eating wild animals could also have exposed early woman and her mate to tularemia (related to bubonic plague), toxoplasmosis, hemorrhagic fevers, and anthrax, alongside gangrene, botulism, and tetanus. And that's to say nothing of the ticks and fleas growing on those animals (potentially carrying plague or sleeping sickness), or the mosquitoes that fed off primates ill with yellow fever, before snacking on human blood.[4]

But while infectious diseases had a dramatic impact on human biology and instincts, and undoubtedly played a role in keeping the original human population in Africa in check, they may not have been the dominant factor. Many diseases were geographically concentrated. And the contagious diseases that were specific to humans couldn't kill too effectively—there were too few humans, too spread out, to allow most deadly conditions to thrive without a reservoir of animal victims to fall back on.[5] Again, hunting and gathering takes a lot more land per person than farming, and early humans would have been constantly on the move. That would have taken them away from areas with parasite-laden feces or mosquitoes gorged on the blood of fellow humans—in turn, reducing the risk of subsequent infection. Any condition that was too deadly would wipe out its hosts before meeting new victims to infect.[6] That suggests it may have been a time of comparatively long natural life expectancy.[7]

Something kept the number of humans planet-wide low. One factor may have been low birth rates among hunter-gatherers. Women who are part of San tribes (the bushmen of Southern Africa) historically gave birth between four and five times, a rate that is similar to Australian aboriginal women.[8] Evidence from other hunter-gatherer communities in Africa—the Kung and the Efe—suggest a woman who lived through her reproductive years would give birth between 2.6 and 4.7 times.[9] That compares to a total fertility rate for Sub-Saharan Africa as a whole that was closer to 7 as recently as 1980. The lower numbers for the Stone Age groups probably reflect a combination of factors that includes a late age of sexual maturity, extended breastfeeding, and considerable movement.[10]

Violence also had a large role in keeping populations in check—perhaps even larger than it did in later ages. In his history of violence, *The Better Angels of Our Nature*, Steven Pinker argues that average pre-civilization rates of violence were higher than anything we've seen since except in *modern* hunter-gatherer societies. Scientists examining prehistoric hunter-gatherer remains in Southern California found that one in five male skeletons showed signs of injury from a projectile like a spear or arrow. At one extreme, Azar Gat of Tel Aviv University concludes his review of hunter-gatherer warfare by suggesting violence accounted for as much as 15 percent of all deaths.[11] Others argue for lower rates of violent deaths overall, and estimates vary considerably across different periods and locations.[12] But the combined result of low birth rates, violence, and the prehistoric infections that did exist was that global populations could be counted in the millions—a tiny fraction of their size today.

The original parasites that preferred *Homo sapiens* had no other option but to live in the tropics—their victim of choice has resided in Africa and nowhere else for most of its time on the planet. Until the rise of civilization sparked the creation of a whole new set of infections, the bacteria, viruses, worms, and other organisms that called humanity home were evolved to complete their life cycle in Africa.

Even today, pathogen diversity (the number of different kinds of microbes in an area that infect humans) remains far higher in the tropics than elsewhere.[13] But because these microbes tend to maim and kill primarily in the developing world, where most people are poor and new drugs to treat the conditions won't make money, they don't attract much in the way of medical research. There's a certain irony that some of humanity's oldest parasitic foes are now grouped together under the moniker "neglected tropical diseases," but that's why.

The control of fire and the invention of clothing allowed for mankind to survive cold winters, and gave us access to the world's temperate zones. By moving to Europe, Asia, and the Americas, we outran some of those parasites. While globalization eventually spread many of the original tropical diseases of Africa to tropical parts of those newly inhabited regions, the long evolution and concentration of human infections in tropical climates is one reason why humans living in temperate zones to the north or south of the tropics remain healthier to this day.[14]

Sometimes when an organism finds itself away from its usual predators and prey, the result is a population explosion, like the Japanese vine kudzu planted in the US, or rabbits in Australia. Humans outside the tropics benefited from this "ecological release." The early years of new occupation in temperate zones like southern Europe and Asia north of the monsoon zone were a period of low infection and rich hunting.[15] That may account for the global spread of humanity in a very brief period. Over about thirty thousand years starting in 40,000 BCE, humans reached every continent but Antarctica.[16]

The expanding human populations that resulted may have played some role in wiping out a number of different large-bodied game animals. South America was home to horses and camels prior to its original human settlement, but they were gone soon after.[17] Even if not, more humans meant more human creativity, which would have been a factor behind the technological innovations that created agriculture.

While plagues don't get a mention in the early chapters of the Bible, once that text reaches Egyptian civilization, it's flooded with stories of pestilence—not only frogs, but boils, lice, flies, and other unknown horrors.[18] That may reflect an underlying historical truth: agriculture and civilization set off a global firestorm of disease.

Even the most inefficient early agriculture was associated with populations per square mile that were ten or twenty times higher than among nomadic groups. And the landscaping and irrigation alongside granaries that accompanied larger-scale farming meant more people had to stay in place—early civilizations enslaved nearby herders to farm their fields.[19] While less movement equals less exposure to new disease pools, the combination of population density and settlement was vital to the growth of infection.

At first, staying in one place for a long time would have been a boost to the traditional afflictions of pre-civilization humans—mosquitoes, for example, would find more people to feed on, and more irrigated and cleared land to live in. And the malaria that used mosquitoes as a vector would spread more rapidly when the chance of the same insect biting, in succession, an infected victim followed by an uninfected one increased by orders of magnitude.[20] A 3000 BCE Egyptian papyrus on medicine contains a reference to "the pest of the year" that may have been malaria, and mummies from the period show evidence of malarial infection.[21]

Bolstering this same point that the more humans are loitering about, the greater the chance of illness: worms excreted onto a village path or into a field or nearby pond were far more likely to wriggle their way into another human than if they'd been defecated in the forest. Microbes that can only survive a small time outside their host, including the bacteria that cause leprosy, typically spread with greater ease in close-packed towns.[22] Finally, the piles of garbage that are the hallmark of any permanent human habitation attract flies, wild dogs, and rats—each with their own disease-spreading potential.

Because civilization involves lots of people and domesticated animals living in close proximity, it also provided the perfect environment for species-hopping infectious killers to spread. Take pigs: they've long had an important role as refuse collectors, demonstrated in Egypt in 2009 when the government took the fateful decision to cull all three hundred thousand of the country's pig population, ostensibly as a measure to prevent the spread of swine flu. Less than a year later, Egypt's parliament was holding a stormy session decrying the policy, which had led to mounting garbage piles across the country. Hamdy el-Sayed, legislator and chairman of the Doctors' Association, called it a "national scandal."[23] But precisely because they eat almost anything, pigs can be a major source of infection themselves. That's likely why both the Jewish and Islamic faiths suggest you shouldn't eat pork. Deuteronomy warns that "the pig, because it has a split hoof, but does not chew the cud; it is unclean for you. You shall neither eat of their flesh nor touch their carcass."

Trichinosis is caused by the pork worm—three millimeters long at their tallest. Thousands of the parasites invade the body of humans unwise enough to eat an infected and undercooked sausage or pork chop. Besides triggering vomiting, diarrhea, and fever, the larvae, as they occupy muscle cells, weaken the victim's heart and diaphragm. Respiratory, heart, or kidney failure related to the parasite can all prove fatal. Pigs themselves pick up the worms by eating garbage containing bits of raw meat or animal remains—or cannibalizing their former farm-mates, or eating a rat that happens to be attracted to the same garbage.[24]

And while sausage lovers may have heard enough already, pigs and humans also share the pork tapeworm. Infected humans can develop cysticercosis, where the worm's larval cysts spread to the brain. The condition can cause seizures, stroke, or death. As many as fifty thousand people still die each year from cysticercosis.[25] While humans were infected by tapeworms long before pig domestication, closer proximity may have increased infection rates.[26]

Over time, and largely within the last few thousand years, a more insidious effect of civilization and domestication emerged: the evolution of new infections. Some diseases of civilization may have evolved from livestock illnesses. Proximity to a dense population of inter-bred domesticated animals presented considerable opportunities for infections to develop and jump species: we've seen that influenza is similar to diseases in pigs and ducks, for example, while diphtheria and rotavirus may have spread from domesticated cattle and sheep (tuberculosis may have jumped the other way, from humans to cows).[27]

Human population density really matters for a number of the most harmful single-species diseases that emerged thanks to civilization. That's because the minimum population required to sustain an infection depends on how rapidly a disease spreads, how deadly it is, and whether infection gives lifelong immunity to survivors.

Microbes that tend to survive in small host populations are those that spread easily, can live outside hosts for a long time, and then live inside their hosts for a long time as well—meaning they kill infrequently and promote no immunity. These were the diseases unique to humans that could best survive the low population densities of pre-civilization. Consider the type of herpes virus that causes cold sores: it has been infecting humans since before they evolved from our ancestor *Homo erectus*. You're quite likely to be living with the virus: about two-thirds of people do. But most of the time cold sores are all it ever causes, and it lives relatively peacefully in your nerve cells until you die.[28]

Compare the torpor of herpes to the relentless-as-Voldemort measles, one of history's biggest murderers. At some point the virus jumped species from cattle to humans. Its first symptoms are a cough and sneezing, which is how it spreads. Only later does the characteristic rash develop. Hosts can die from complications related to a swollen brain caused by encephalitis, diarrhea and dehydration, or pneumonia.

The first time that a disease like measles or smallpox arrives, it rips through the entire population, infecting widely and killing off those particularly susceptible—because of factors like age, malnutrition, or genetic variation. But the survivors become immune, often for life. And if most of the population has been exposed, that creates "herd immunity": the number of potential victims has shrunk, and so the chance that a coughed-out measles virus reaches a non-immune host drops. If that chance falls far enough so that the average person with measles infects less than one new victim, the epidemic eventually dies out.

Sadly, however, newborns don't inherit measles immunity. As a new generation of potential hosts grows, herd immunity fails and measles returns to ravage the population of previously unexposed children. A measles victim is likely to pass on the infection to twelve or more people in an unexposed population, and that means for herd immunity to defeat a measles outbreak, more than 92 percent of the community needs to be individually immune. In turn, that suggests only a few years of new births is required before the proportion of immune people drops below the share necessary to preserve herd immunity and measles can strike again.

The estimate is that to survive and re-infect later generations, measles needs at least five hundred thousand people living in close proximity—otherwise it dies out. And only with an even larger connected population does a disease like measles change from an epidemic (appearing in waves as a new generation of victims grows large enough) to being endemic (always present, infecting the young and previously unexposed). Measles needs large civilizations if it is to survive and thrive.

Three thousand years elapsed between the first evidence of domestic plants and livestock and the beginnings of permanent towns, and about three thousand more counted down before the emergence of the first cities with tributary lands, like Ur and Kish.[29] Even these cities began as homes to only ten to twenty thousand people—simply not large enough to sustain a disease like measles.[30] But as civilizations grew, measles and smallpox both jumped species to make a permanent home in humans.[31]

And in larger populations, these new diseases became part of the mundane background of life. The history of smallpox in Japan provides an illustration. By the 1600s, the disease was endemic in Japan's urban areas. Suffering and recovering from smallpox became a significant part of the ritual celebrating a child's growth. But in outlying islands with small populations and limited connectivity, the disease remained a periodic, epidemic visitor. And behavior toward smallpox was notably different. Visitors from Japan's central regions were surprised that islanders would flee from the infection and quarantine victims, often abandoning family members.

According to historian Akihito Suzuki "these behaviors caused emotions ranging from curious bewilderment to moral condemnation of . . . an unthinkable barbarity" among visitors from the city.[32] But the different behavior has an utterly rational component. In endemic environments, smallpox exposure is going to happen—it's only a matter of when. A level of fatalism is sensible under the circumstances. In communities where a disease only reappears every few years, it might be possible to avoid catching it.

Even if these different reactions may make sense, they probably give us a skewed sense of history. We tend to view irregular, concentrated mortality differently from daily, small-scale mortality (think of deaths from plane crashes versus car crashes—the first garner more attention, the second kill more people). And we're dulled into inaction by frequent association: how else to explain the fact that most with access to the seasonal flu vaccine don't get it despite the flu's killing more than half a million people per year worldwide.[33] On the other hand, people *notice* epidemics and pandemics, calling them plagues. Potential victims run from them. Chroniclers record them and poets bewail them. Sometimes they help end empires. Everyday endemic infection is hardly worth a stanza, let alone flight.

Nonetheless, over the millennia it was the regular, endemic infections (like malaria and—in larger communities—smallpox and measles) that killed greater numbers than dramatic plagues and pestilences. Day-to-day unfriendly local infections felled a third or more people before they reached adulthood. And, in the end, they had the larger role in shaping societies and economies.

We can see the massive health burden that is created when previously unexposed populations are presented with the full diversity of agro-urban disease. An analysis of 238 recently contacted Brazilian indigenous societies from the Amazon basin suggests their population numbers fell an average of 43 percent in the nine years after sustained contact with outsiders from the connected villages and cities of modern Brazil.[34]

Again, archaeologists have dug up skeletons from peoples who made the transition from hunting to agriculture, and the bones of the agricultural groups are in worse shape than those of their hunter forebears. The bones have lesions in them: signs of infection. Anemia—low oxygen-carrying capacity in the blood, often linked to infection—frequently leaves its mark in spongy bones. And the teeth have low levels of enamel, associated with an unhealthy childhood.

But the liabilities of the agricultural lifestyle don't stop there. Archaeologists with the stomach to study preserved human feces (coprolites) find more intestinal parasites preserved within them as human groups move through the agricultural revolution.

Alongside more infection risk, people in early civilizations experienced worse nutrition. The field-tending masses became more reliant on a few staple crops and ate less protein. We know broadly what their diet must have looked like because of its likely similarity to the diet of today's very poorest people. Take the Aboubakar family of Breidjing Refugee Camp in Eastern Chad, interviewed by Peter Menzel and Faith D'Aluisio a few years ago for their book *Hungry Planet*. The family benefited from the fact that relief agencies were supplying them with staple foods, but their meals were still immensely monotonous. The Aboubakars ate forty-four pounds of grain—mostly sorghum—each week. They ate five pounds of beans, two and a half pounds of vegetables, alongside a couple of quarts of cooking oil and some sugar. But the six family members split just nine ounces of goat and six ounces of fish for the week. The only fruit was five limes (less than one each). They ate no dairy at all.

At least this variety of calories was sufficient to stave off wasting—many poor people outside refugee camps do even worse. Take this description of daily life from a person living in poverty in Vietnam: "In the mornings, eat sweet potatoes, work. At lunch, go without. In the evenings, eat sweet potatoes, sleep."[35]

In the earliest civilizations (again, as with the poorest people alive today), the meat that people did get to eat was more likely to be infested with the types of parasite which enjoy living in humans for part of their life cycle. And malnutrition and infection reinforce each other. If you don't get enough vitamins and minerals, you're more likely to get sick. For example, vitamin A deficiency increases the risk of diarrhea, malaria, and measles, while zinc deficiency reduces the overall effectiveness of the immune system.[36] And parasites, in particular, drain nutrients from human hosts—many worms absorb them directly from inside the intestine.[37] Over the millennia, people literally shrank under the combined influence of infection and malnutrition—women by as much as four centimeters on average from their prehistoric height.

The process didn't reverse until very recently: the depths of human stature probably weren't reached until the hellhole cities of the Industrial Revolution.[38] In 1841, Liverpool saw an *average* life expectancy of less than twenty-six years—that's at or below the rate estimated for life expectancy in tropical Africa at the time.[39] In 1842, the average age of death in Manchester was just seventeen years old for laborers. That compared to fifty-two for gentry in the countryside area of Rutland and thirty-eight for rural laborers. A mean age of death of seventeen is considerably lower than estimates for hunter-gatherers in prehistory.[40]

The effects of civilization were particularly grim for women.[41] The mélange of infections produced by urbanization and agriculture demanded high birth rates to keep up with the high rates of childhood mortality.[42] Accordingly, the average woman for most of recorded history spent a considerable proportion of her life from adolescence to menopause pregnant or breastfeeding.[43]

In turn, that often reduced women's autonomy. Many Stone Age groups saw some level of equality between the sexes in terms of roles and decision-making. But the Code of Hammurabi, sixth king of Babylon, suggests how times changed with civilization. Hammurabi, who ruled Mesopotamia around 3,770 years ago, created one of the earliest known sets of laws. These precepts treated women only a little better than property: "If a man strike a freeborn woman so that she lose her unborn child, he shall pay ten shekels for her loss. . . . If the woman die, his daughter shall be put to death."[44]

The range of diseases that civilization enabled was effective in keeping human population below the carrying capacity of the land.

The Danish economist Ester Boserup challenged Malthus's ideas about land limits and food supply in her 1965 book *The Conditions of Agricultural Growth.*[45] She pointed out that a population increase may expand the land area used for agriculture, but more significantly, it leads to intensification—producing more food from the same land. One simple change was to redirect land being used for pasture toward growing crops.[46] And she notes that techniques to increase the amount of food per acre, like crop rotation, were known long before they were widely introduced.[47] Through most of history and in most places, Boserup suggested, neither technological barriers nor lack of land prevented greater output.

Earth scientist Jed Kaplan and colleagues suggest that less than one-*half* of the land currently used for food production was used in 1600 and less than one-*third* in 100 CE.[48] It is true that making more of the land available takes more work—sometimes brutally hard work, and that risks malnutrition. Again, some land couldn't be cultivated without innovations, including heavy plows and irrigation. Nonetheless, it seems clear that throughout most of history the number of humans on earth fluctuated far below the maximum possible.

Instead, we should probably thank (or blame) the regulatory mechanism of infection for limiting populations. As the number of people grew, population density drove up disease rates. This thinning mechanism was, in most places, probably the most powerful check on the number of people, particularly during the centuries that humans have been farmers.

Evidence of the relative role of different Malthusian checks is provided by what we know of the history of mass starvation. Cormac Ó Gráda in his *Famine: A Short History* provides data and descriptions of some of the world's worst famines. Two points are worth making: first, most are associated with war or a run of bad weather (usually drought, less often rains and floods). It's not that the usual productive capacity of the land comes close to subsistence, it's that an extreme shock drives productivity far closer to or even below subsistence. Second, even the most deadly of famines he lists—Ireland in 1740–41 and 1846–52, China in 1877–79 and 1959–61, Cambodia in 1975–79—killed a maximum of "only" 15 to 25 million people, or 13 percent of the population. Pandemics like the Black Death managed far worse over far larger areas, and endemic diseases like smallpox take a far larger regular toll over the long term.[49]

Again, the degree to which population is driven up or down by infection—as opposed to malnutrition and starvation—is demonstrated by the recorded health history of the rich. Wealthy people can afford better diets. And yet Walter Scheidel's study of Roman emperors who died natural deaths as well as senators and their families suggests life expectancies at birth for the elite were less than thirty years.[50] This was a group famed for its dining habits. The Roman cookbook *De Re Coquinaria* lists recipes for pheasant, goose, peacock, chicken, flamingo, parrot, crane, duck, wood pigeon, squab, figpecker, partridge, turtle dove, woodcock, and ostrich, to mention some of the birds alone. Full stomachs didn't seem to confer much longevity.

Throughout most of history, to keep population-dense cities like Rome occupied took a constant stream of rural migrants—because urban populations couldn't produce enough children to keep up with death rates. Especially in early civilizations, that migration was rarely voluntary. James Scott argues in his *Against the Grain* that ancient states "replenished their population by wars of capture and by buying slaves on a large scale from barbarians who specialized in the trade."[51]

The largest cities drew in new victims from hundreds of miles of hinterlands and boasted comparatively advanced sanitation, but still they couldn't be sustained over the long term. If war or imperial collapse removed the power and ability to attract migrants, urban populations could rapidly collapse. According to Tertius Chandler, the population of Athens halved between 430 and 100 BCE as the city was eclipsed by Rome, and in turn the population of Rome fell by nearly 90 percent between 100 CE and 600 CE as the empire began to fall apart.[52]

To be absolutely clear, most of history has still seen Malthusian outcomes at a local level: as populations rise, average incomes and consumption fall. But it appears that only at times of crisis, sometimes linked to changing climate, has lack of food become the binding constraint to population numbers. Ester Boserup was right: it wasn't shortage of land. What kept populations low and dispersed was a high death rate driven by infection. And when infectious death declined in the nineteenth and twentieth centuries, population, urbanization, intensification, land use, *and* prosperity all climbed to historically unprecedented levels worldwide.

CHAPTER THREE

Trade Merges Disease Pools

. . . a pestilence, by which the whole human race came near to being annihilated.

—Procopius

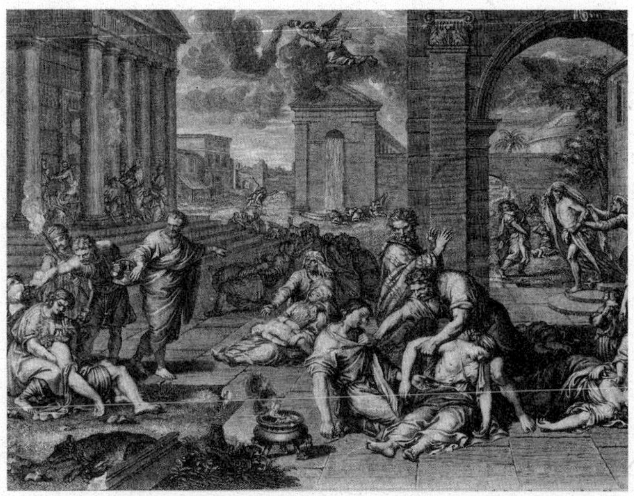

The plague of the Israelites—supposedly a heavenly punishment for running an improper census.

(Credit: *The Plague of the Israelites*. Engraving by E. G. Petit, 172–, after P. Mignard. Wellcome Library, no. 6346i)

Agriculture and cities are sedentary—people largely stay where they are to manage fields, markets, and temples. And, historically, that created the need for trade: if you couldn't move to where the goods were, the goods would have to move instead. James Scott has suggested that the early state centers in Mesopotamia traded for wood, leather, obsidian, copper, tin, gold, silver, and honey.[1] But with the goods (and even more so, the slaves) that were transported by boat, horse, and porter came the diseases of foreign lands. Add the migration of troops in warfare and the first steps on the pathway to a global disease pool had begun.[2]

Ancient Greek city states paid a high price for this growing connectedness. They were particularly susceptible to foreign diseases because they were so reliant on trade. The country's thin limestone soil received little rain, so its population clustered on the coasts, where the sea offered sustenance. To supplement their diet of fish, Athenians imported grain from the Crimea, Sicily, and Alexandria. In some years, as much as 3 million bushels—more than forty Olympic swimming pools' worth—were imported through the Black Sea alone.[3]

The plague of Athens was one of the earliest reliably recorded pandemics. According to the chronicler Thucydides, who suffered from the plague himself, it spread through North Africa and then invaded Athens in 430 BCE. Despite Thucydides's detailed description, argument rages over what the disease was—one strong candidate is typhoid; Ebola is also a contender.[4] But we don't recognize the collection of symptoms described by Thucydides as a single modern infection, perhaps because it has evolved since then.

> People in good health were all of a sudden attacked by violent heats in the head, and redness and inflammation in the eyes, the inward parts, such as the throat or tongue, becoming bloody and emitting an unnatural and fetid breath. These symptoms were followed by sneezing and hoarseness, after which the pain soon reached the chest, and produced a hard cough. When it fixed in the stomach, it upset it; and discharges of bile of every kind named by physicians ensued. . . . The patient could not bear to have on him clothing or linen even of the very lightest description; or indeed to be otherwise than stark naked. . . . They succumbed . . . in most cases, on the seventh or eighth day to the internal inflammation. . . . But if they passed this stage, and the disease descended further into the bowels, inducing a violent ulceration there accompanied by severe diarrhoea, this brought on a weakness which was generally fatal.[5]

In part thanks to the plague, Athens lost its war against neighboring Sparta. Not for the last time, disease was a force for considerable social and economic upheaval. The great academic Arnold Toynbee, author of the twelve-volume *Study of History*, was overwrought on the subject, but he saw the glories of democratic Athens giving way to an authoritarian utopianism bolstered by the intellectual backing of the philosophers Plato and Aristotle:

> In Plato's Utopias and Aristotle's alike . . . the aim is not the happiness of the individual but the stability of the community. Plato . . . advocates a general censorship over "dangerous thought" that has its latter-day parallels in the regulations of Communist Russia, National-Socialist Germany, Fascist Italy and Shintoist Japan.[6]

We will see the type of authoritarian control and xenophobia of which Toynbee accused the Greek philosophers frequently accompany disease outbreaks up to and including border closing responses to the Ebola outbreaks of 2014 and the fast-moving Covid pandemic in 2020.

In the same century as Athens was weakened by plague, the Roman historian Livy reports his city was fighting the Aequi and Volscians when an outbreak struck:

> The violence of the epidemic was aggravated by the crowding into the city of the country people and their cattle through fear of raids. . . . Their being brought into contact with each other in ordinary intercourse helped to spread the disease. The mortality in Rome through the epidemic was not less than that of the allies through the sword. . . . The Senate, deprived of all human aid, bade the people betake themselves to prayers.[7]

Infection did not stop the rise of the city state, perhaps in part because it assailed the young republic and its enemies alike, and involved local infections rather than new pandemic imports. But as Rome grew and conquered distant lands, this would change.

By the time Julius Caesar dismantled what was left of the Roman Republic, the city's empire was one of the biggest the world had seen. More than 50 million people lived under Caesar's rule, stretching from the Atlantic coast of Gaul to the headwaters of the Nile. Frederick Cartwright, a medical historian, describes "the makings of disaster":

> A vast hinterland hiding unknown secrets, among them the micro-organisms of foreign disease; troops who attacked into that hinterland and were attacked by the inhabitants; free transit by ship or along roads specially built for speedy travel; at the center a concentrated population living a highly civilized life yet lacking the most rudimentary means of combating infection.[8]

Roman merchants benefited from the Empire's central highway, the Mediterranean Sea, which allowed for dramatically faster travel than even Rome's roads. And common merchandise included slaves (more than 1 million from Caesar's Gallic Wars alone) that were the perfect vessels for moving infection.[9]

The merchants traveled even farther than did Rome's troops. They set up a trading station near modern Pondicherry in India in CE 14. Within a century, thousands of Romans may have been traveling to India each year. Pliny the Elder, adviser to Emperor Vespasian in the first century CE, noted extensive Roman imports from across the Indian Ocean. In an attack on trade deficits with Asia that might sound familiar today, he complained that "India drains more than 50 million sesterces a year from our Empire."[10] It was a sum greater than Caesar had demanded in tribute from Gaul after his conquest.

Caesar himself gave Cleopatra an outfit of Chinese silk reportedly so gauzy as to be see-through, setting a fashion trend that swept Rome.[11] In 160 CE, Roman ambassadors traveled through Egypt and Ethiopia, across the Indian Ocean and north to Vietnam by sea, and then overland to Luoyang in Han China. Chinese chroniclers suggest they brought elephant tusks, rhinoceros horns, and turtle shells as gifts. The visit cemented the relationship of the world's two greatest empires, between them home to half of the people on earth.[12]

There is a detailed description of the Roman Empire, known as Da Qin, from China. *The Peoples of the West*, published in the third century CE, reported:

> The kingdom of Da Qin . . . has more than four hundred smaller cities and towns. It extends several thousand *li* in all directions. The king has his capital close to the mouth of a river. The outer walls of the city are made of stone. . . . [They have] a tradition of amazing conjuring. They can produce fire from their mouths, bind and then free themselves, and juggle twelve balls with extraordinary skill. . . .
>
> The people cultivate the five grains, and they raise horses, mules, donkeys, camels and silkworms. This country produces fine linen. They make gold and silver coins. One gold coin is equal to ten silver coins. They have fine brocaded cloth that is said to be made from the down of "water-sheep." . . . They regularly make a profit by obtaining Chinese silk, unraveling it, and making fine silk damasks.[13]

For all the titillation that the silk trade allowed Caesar, it also carried infection risk. Just as Roman merchants arrived in China in 166 CE, what might have been smallpox reached back to Europe, perhaps brought on its final leg by troops campaigning in Mesopotamia. Hammering the area just as the climate was cooling (reducing yields and, consequently, nutrition levels), that disease killed more than one in four people in parts of the empire.[14]

Contemporary accounts report that the Antonine plague (named after Emperor Marcus Aurelius Antoninus) spread from Persia to the Rhine, killing enough people that whole cities were abandoned and wars ceased for lack of healthy armies.

This was the first year that German tribes—the Marcomanni and the Quadi—broke through the Roman defensive positions on the border of the empire, a sign of things to come as Rome was struck again and again by epidemics.[15] Around 250 CE, another in a series of plagues killed as many as half of the population of some cities as well as an emperor.[16] Historian Kyle Harper reports that the Cyprian plague, as it has become known, involved violent vomiting and diarrhea, putrefaction of extremities, and victims becoming deaf and blind—which suggests it might have been a hemorrhagic fever in the same family as Ebola. He also notes that the plague coincided with German tribes breaking across the Rhine to devastate Gaul and penetrate both Spain and Northern Italy; Goths striking at Greece, Macedonia, and parts of the empire in Asia; and the Parthians conquering Roman territory in Mesopotamia and Syria.[17]

Adding to the burden of a cycle of plagues, the most serious strain of malaria, falciparum, spread slowly up the Italian peninsula over the thousand-year life of the republic and empire. It reached Rome around 400 BCE and Venice by 750 CE. As it spread to previously unaffected regions, it would kill off considerable numbers of the most vulnerable. One of the largest ancient Roman infant cemeteries discovered dates to about 450 CE. It's in Lugnano in Teverina, seventy miles from Rome, and contains forty-seven babies, all buried in the same summer, nearly half of which were premature. Falciparum malaria frequently causes miscarriages in previously unexposed pregnant women. The oldest child found on the site was a girl aged two or three years old. Her hands and feet were weighed down under stones and tiles, perhaps to prevent the demon disease from escaping to cause further destruction. DNA tests confirm she had malaria.[18]

But it was a pandemic that finished off the empire. Justinian, who ruled from 527 CE to 565 CE, was the last emperor to semi-successfully stitch back together many of the lands that had been ruled in Rome's heyday, including Italy, much of Spain, and North Africa to the Atlantic. His contemporary biographer Procopius wrote glowing official accounts of these victories as well as a considerably less flattering secret history that described his boss as "an unnatural mixture of folly and wickedness . . . deceitful, devious, false, hypocritical, two-faced, cruel, skilled in dissembling his thought."[19] On the subject of violence, "sooner could one number, I fancy, the sands of the sea than the men this Emperor murdered," declared the biographer. Incessant and barbaric war sparked by Justinian depopulated large areas, says Procopius: "The whole earth ran red with the blood of nearly all the Romans and the barbarians."[20]

But alongside the human violence came death by infection. In his *History of the Wars*, Procopius describes the terror that affected the period, beginning in 542 CE: "a pestilence, by which the whole human race came near to being annihilated." This was an outbreak of *Yersinia pestis*, the plague of the Black Death, paying its first significant visit to Mediterranean shores in recorded history. (It may have previously visited Europe to ravage substantial Neolithic settlements linked by the new technology of the wheel five thousand years before.)[21]

The disease we typically refer to as "the" plague usually spreads via infected rats and fleas. Fleas pass on the plague through a bite, and when their host dies they hop off to find sustenance elsewhere, taking the bacillus with them. The fever that heralds onset appeared to be nothing significant, suggested Procopius. But not many days later, a "swelling developed; and this took place not only . . . below the abdomen, but also inside the armpit, and in some cases also beside the ears, and at different points on the thighs." The condition progresses through high fever, muscle cramps and seizures, sometimes with vomiting. Parts of the body develop gangrene as the host begins rotting from within. Unlucky victims—often the majority without modern medical treatment—go on to coma and death.

The deadly nature of the plague helps keep it local—unless humans move it. As William Bernstein observed in his history of global commerce, "plague is a disease of trade." To transport the bacillus to the next stop on the caravan route or port, "the human, rodent and insect hosts must pass quickly across the seas and steppes."[22] Camels may have played a vital role in transporting the plague bacillus over distances—they can catch the disease and even infect humans directly if they're slaughtered and eaten.[23] But the plague still needs a concentrated population of rats and fleas to help it spread rapidly in new locales—and cities along ancient trade routes provided suitable conditions for that.

The outbreak of plague that spread across the empire originated in Asia. It was first recorded reaching Roman territory in Pelusium, which sat on the east side of the Nile delta.[24] That was a scant 160 miles down the coast from Alexandria, to which plague quickly spread. Alexandria was the second largest city in the Mediterranean and a port that sent grain from the rich fields of the Nile floodplains across the Roman Empire. In turn, that meant the city teamed with cosmopolitan rats, which boarded ships bound for Constantinople, Rome, and beyond, well supplied with food. Without sea trade, the bacillus might not have made it much past Pelusium. But Alexandria's rodents helped carry the plague to the ends of the empire.[25]

Procopius was in Constantinople at the time the plague reached the imperial capital and reports that the towers of the city walls were piled up with dead for lack of burial places. Again, the chronicler suggests survivors became wanton, "surpassing themselves in villainy and in lawlessness of every sort."[26] Nearly half of the city's half-million strong population may have perished.[27] (It should be noted Procopius remained privately of the opinion that the emperor was worse than the plague: "Some never were taken by the disease, and others recovered after it had smitten them. But this man, not one of all the Romans could escape . . . as if he were a second pestilence sent from heaven.")[28]

In 543, within a year of striking Constantinople, plague had reached Arles in Southern Gaul. And the disease reappeared again and again over the next thirty years. Out of 26 million of Justinian's subjects, as many as 4 million died in the first two years and 5 million more within the sixty years that followed. Cities shrank to towns, towns to villages, and many villages disappeared altogether. Land under cultivation across the empire as much as halved.[29]

The plague helped unravel Justinian's re-knitting of empire. The army that could be supported by a diminished economy was one-third the size of that before the plague struck. Justinian's son, Justin II, saw the Lombards occupy Italy, the Slavs take land throughout the Balkans, and the Avars settle on the Danube. From a rebounding Mediterranean civilization in the pre-plague period and the attempts to reconstitute the glory that was Rome in its heyday, within decades of the first Plague of Justinian the empire was shrinking toward a rump around Constantinople.

The Mediterranean region soon became a battle zone between Christians in the northwest and a new religion from the southeast—Islam. In 545 and 546, plague ripped through Mesopotamia, returning again and again to weaken the Persian Empire. Then in 569, Abyssinians fell back from the walls of Mecca thanks to pestilence.[30] The Abyssinians were there, so the story goes, because an Arab chief from Mecca had defecated in a new cathedral constructed in Abyssinia. But their forces, led by an elephant, were met by the prayers of Mecca's inhabitants. The elephant kneeled before the city while Allah sent birds each carrying stones the size of lentils to drop on the invaders. All sixty thousand struck were killed. This was in the year—perhaps even on the day—of the birth of the prophet Muhammad.

Islam survived and subsequently prospered in a largely plague-free Saudi peninsula after both Persia and the Roman Empire were crippled by plague. By 630 CE, Muhammad's armies controlled all of Arabia, shutting off the sea route to the Indian Ocean. Within generations, the land route of the silk road would be closed, too. Exchange in silk, spices, and (probably) microbes all shrank back.[31]

The "Muslim quarantine," although far from a complete halt to trading and exchange, helped keep Europe safe from renewed infection from the south and east. Forests spread between populated areas within Europe, slowing travel and further reducing trade. The greatly diminished movement of people within the former Roman Empire insulated populations against new and old diseases alike. Older people who had experienced earlier waves of plague and other infections (and lived to tell the tale) were immune. And circumstances were against diseases of density: the number of people in Europe declined from 70 million at the height of the Roman Empire to 25 million by 700 CE. Urban populations (the most favorable hosts for infection) shrank from half a million in Rome to twenty-five times smaller in the largest cities of 800.[32]

The remaining population was likely to have been better nourished and so more resistant to disease, the result of retreating to the most productive land for crops and using some of the rest for livestock. Justinian tried to freeze prices and wages, complaining that people had abandoned themselves to avarice, but the labor shortage gave farmworkers new leverage. The practice of using slaves on farms in Spain and Italy died out, replaced by the feudal system of serfs who owed loyalty and labor to a lord in return for land.[33] And the Black Death disappeared.

Over the next centuries, lowered infection levels thanks to low population densities and restricted trade created the potential for renewed population growth in Europe. The weather also improved—enough for Britain to start producing wine (although chroniclers are silent on its quality). From the low point of the Dark Ages to 1300, populations tripled. Forests and pastures were converted back to cropland.[34] Cities including Milan and Paris climbed toward two hundred thousand residents.

As the pestilences of the Roman Empire presaged the plague at its end, so did sickness and strife come before the hammer fall of the Black Death. For perhaps the first and only time in Northern European history, the Malthusian constraint of land availability threatened to become a major factor in determining death rates. The consequences of a bad growing season could be devastating. And when a series of bad seasons struck in a row, as they did from 1315 to 1322, deaths climbed into the hundreds of thousands across the continent.[35]

As early as 1316, reports John Kelly in his history of the period *The Great Mortality*, "as food grew costlier, people ate bird dung, family pets, mildewed wheat, corn and finally, in desperation, they ate one another." Just as climate change may have helped create a weakened population toward the end of the Roman Empire, so it did in the fourteenth century.

And sources for continent-spanning epidemics were available once again, because long-distance trade had burgeoned. In 1206, the tribes of an obscure nomadic kingdom gathered at Karakorum in Mongolia to elect a new khan (leader). His name was Chinghiz, and he set his people on a road of conquest that, within two decades, left the great majority of the Eurasian landmass under their control. The Great Khan and his subordinates ruled territory from Eastern Europe to the Pacific, excluding only India, Arabia, and parts of Southeast Asia.

For all the fear generated by "a peril impending and palpably approaching" (as Pope Alexander IV put it in an appeal for Christian unity against the invaders), some Europeans saw the opportunities presented by the world's newest and greatest superpower.[36] In 1260, Niccolo and Maffeo Polo set off from the Venetian colony of Sudak on the Crimean peninsula to trade at the capital of Berke Khan, lord of the Western Tartars, to the north of the Caspian Sea. The Polos ended up at the court of his kinsman Kublai Khan in China.

Marco Polo, Niccolo's son, accompanied his father on a return trip a few years later. He recounted the many quality goods produced along the route: the best goshawks in the world in Georgia, Persian steeds exported to India alongside the finest asses in the world, pearls pierced in Baghdad imported from India and sent on to Europe. He describes Tabriz: "a market for merchandise from India and Baghdad, from Mosul and Hormuz, and from many other places," where Latin merchants came to buy merchandise. Hormuz itself was regularly visited by Indian merchants bringing spices, precious stones, elephant tusks, and cloth of silk and gold. And Kashgar was "the starting point from which many merchants set out to market their wares all over the world."[37]

Seventy-five years later, the poet Petrarch was living in Venice and described the ships voyaging east:

> "If you had seen this vessel you would have said it was not a boat but a mountain swimming in the surface of the sea. . . . It is set-

> ting out for the river Don . . . as far as our ships can sail on the Black Sea, but many of those on board will disembark and journey on, not stopping until they have crossed the Ganges . . . then on to furthest China.[38]

There was so much to trade, and under the united control of the Mongol Empire, that trade was considerably more straightforward than previously when it had been necessary to work through the middlemen of the Middle East. As in Roman times the trade was unequal: while cloth and iron utensils went east, they weren't nearly enough to pay for the silk, spices, skins, wood, salt, grain, and slaves that flowed west. The balance was made up in bullion.[39]

In passing, Marco Polo had mentioned something about the diet of herdsmen he met along his way: "They live on meat and milk and game and on Pharaoh's rats, which are abundant everywhere in the steppes."[40] By Pharaoh's rats, Polo probably meant marmots. The Tarbagan marmot can be an animal reservoir for the Black Death.

In his classic text *Plagues and Peoples*, historian William McNeill suggests that in the midst of a dry spell, herdsmen moved en masse into the northern steppe, where the Tarbagan marmot makes its home. This may have been the starting point of the Great Mortality—the return of the Black Death. By 1331, a mystery epidemic killed as many as nine out of ten in Hopei, Northeast China. The next year, the Great Khan Jijaghatu Toq Temur, ruler of Mongolia, died of a strange new illness along with his sons. By 1338, Kirgizia, in the northwest corner of China, was seeing an outbreak of pestilence recorded on thousands of gravestones of the afflicted.

We'll see that McNeill's version of events in East Asia is disputed. But eight years after the Kirgizia pestilence, Russian chroniclers report a plague arriving on the western shore of the Caspian Sea. And a year after that, it reached the Black Sea.

In 1347, the plague struck a Mongol army besieging the Genoese trading outpost of Caffa, today the town of Feodosiya in Crimea. Twenty years later, Gabriele de Mussi, a notary in the town of Piacenza, Italy, told the story as he heard it. The Mongols (or Tartars, as he calls them)

> "besieged the trapped Christians there for almost three years. . . . But behold, the whole army was affected by a disease which overran the Tartars and killed thousands upon thousands every day. It was as though arrows were raining down from heaven to strike and crush the Tartars' arrogance. All medical advice and attention was useless; the Tartars died as soon as the signs of disease appeared on their bodies; swellings on the armpit and groin caused by coagulating humours, followed by a putrid fever.[41]

Despite the lifting of the siege because of the hideous death toll among the besiegers, occupants of the city did no better. Whether it was by way of fleas carried on rats from besieger to besieged or through direct contact with fleas from Mongol cadavers flung over the walls, the defenders were soon infected themselves. Those who could, fled the mystery illness by sea. As they traveled west, docking at Constantinople, Messina, Sardinia, Genoa, and Marseilles, they may have brought the pestilence with them—at least it followed on later ships from other Crimean ports.[42]

The poet Petrarch's friend, the writer Boccaccio, lived through the plague in Florence and describes early symptoms that match Procopius's description from eight hundred years before. "It first betrayed itself by the emergence of certain tumors in the groin or the armpits, some of which grew as large as a common apple, others as an egg." And the disease spread "despite all that human wisdom and forethought could devise to avert it, as the cleansing of the city from many impurities by officials appointed for the purpose, the refusal of entrance to all sick folk, and the adoption of many precautions for the preservation of health; despite also humble supplications addressed to God."[43]

Petrarch himself, who'd moved from Venice back to his childhood home of Avignon, wrote that "in the year 1348, one that I deplore, we were deprived not only of our friends but of peoples throughout the world. . . . When at any time has such a thing been seen or spoken of? Has what happened in these years ever been read about: empty houses, derelict cities, ruined estates, fields strewn with cadavers, a horrible and vast solitude encompassing the whole world."[44]

Petrarch described his home town Avignon as "the most dismal, crowded and turbulent in existence, a sink overflowing with all of the gathered filth of the world." That suggests it was probably home to a considerable quantity of rats.[45] It was also one of the best connected cities in Europe, and temporary home of the Catholic pope.

Ecologists José Gómez and Miguel Verdú studied which areas were hardest hit by the Black Death, finding that the loss of life in most cities averaged one-half of inhabitants. And (as is usually the case with pandemics) those cities that were more connected, on trade and pilgrimage routes, were more severely affected. They suffered constantly renewed outbreaks. Avignon saw death rates as high as 70 percent.[46]

Pope Clement bought the city a new cemetery to deal with the rising pile of bodies, but it was soon filled with eleven thousand of them, so he simply consecrated the Rhone River as a burial site. Every morning, hundreds of corpses were flung into the river.

As with previous pandemics, one of the signs of a civilization overburdened was the abandoning of suitable reverence for the dead. Petrarch wrote that "wherever I turn my frightened eyes, their gaze is troubled by continual funerals: the churches groan encumbered with biers, and, without last respects, the corpses of the noble and the commoner lie in confusion alongside each other."[47]

That said, while the poet bemoaned "fields strewn with cadavers,"[48] the contemporary descriptions of social breakdown often aped Thucydides's story of the plague of Athens closely enough to suggest chroniclers may have been writing what felt right to say as much as what had happened.[49] And the broader evidence is of remarkably little social disruption.

There *were* exceptions: the worst were deadly outbreaks of anti-Semitism, as we'll see. But, sadly, it hadn't taken the death of as much as half the European population to spark previous violence against Jews in 1146, 1189, 1204, 1217, 1288, 1298, or 1321.[50] Anti-Semitic attacks were an endemic evil throughout much of European history, not a unique sign of a sense of end-times.

Again, in 1349, flagellants wove through towns singing and scourging themselves in repentance, threatening religious authority. On July 8, they entered Strasbourg. All but one man lay face-down on the ground, while the sole standing flagellant brought out his scourge—a whip with many leather tails, each knotted around a thorn at its end. The leader stood over one of the prone brothers and whipped his back with the scourge, saying "Rise up from the cleansing pain and stay away from sin from now on." The first man to feel the lash now joined the leader in taking up the scourge, and the two flagellants moved together to their next kinsman and whipped him, repeating "Rise up from the cleansing pain and stay away from sin from now on." And so they went on around the circle, with each standing brother joining in whipping those who came after, until all two hundred flagellants were upright, walking in a circle, whipping themselves with scourges.

But for all of the drama, the movement quickly petered out. The pope issued a decree against the flagellants in October 1349, and in a case of the punishment fitting the crime perhaps a little too well, a number were condemned to be flogged by priests before the altar of St. Peter's in Rome.[51]

If evidence is needed of the resilience of social order in the face of even the most incredible stress, it is this: people lived through the Black Death, as they lived through epidemics of measles and smallpox—or the Blitz in the Second World War, the 9/11 attacks, or floods in New Orleans—largely *without* resorting to Hobbesian misrule. For all cable news and zombie movies would like to pretend that we're always only a step away from mass hysteria, it's just hardly ever true. The Black Death struck in the midst of the Hundred Years War between England and France, but provoked a cessation of hostilities that lasted only half a year.[52] Edward III's arguable claim to the throne of France couldn't be stopped by the mere death of half of his countrymen.

And, in a world where most people lived largely self-sufficiently and near subsistence, a massive demographic catastrophe had a relatively small short-term impact on the economy. While Sienna's courts and cloth industry all closed down during the height of the plague between June and August 1348, for example, government and the markets were functioning again by the fall of that year.[53]

Mass death in a Malthusian world did eventually have an impact on society and incomes across Western Europe, but that impact was to make the laborers who remained a little better off. In 1349, the English government issued the Ordinance of Labourers. It was prefaced by a justification by King Edward III: "Because a great part of the people, and especially of workmen and servants, late died of the pestilence, many seeing the necessity of masters, and great scarcity of servants, will not serve unless they may receive excessive wages."[54] Workers were using limited supply to demand increased payment, just as they had after the plague of Justinian.

And echoing Justinian's response, Edward III tried to stop that, along with people moving to new jobs or charging higher prices. But just as Justinian's ordinance had been eight centuries earlier, the law was at best partially effective. Suddenly wealthy artisans started eating and dressing better. So the government tried banning that, too. The English sumptuary law passed in 1363 complained of "the Outrageous and Excessive Apparel of divers People, against their Estate and Degree, to the great Destruction and Impoverishment of all the Land." It set down strict rules on who could wear and eat what: servants were to have "Flesh or Fish, and the Remnant [of] other Victuals, as of Milk, Butter, and Cheese" only once a day.

Expensive labor once again made people search for labor-saving devices as they had after the plague of Justinian. Gutenberg's printing technology replaced skilled copyists with the wood and metal of the press, new salting methods allowed smaller fishing crews to stay at sea longer, better pumps drained deeper mines, saving the labor of opening a new one.[55] And in Western Europe, the feudal system that grew up after Justinian's plague to replace farming based on slave labor finally collapsed in turn as a result of the Black Death.[56]

Nico Voigtländer of UCLA and Hans-Joachim Voth, an economist at University Pompeu Fabra in Barcelona, suggest the Black Death wasn't just a boon for laborers in general but also for women in particular. The sudden drop in farm labor encouraged techniques that used less labor on marginal land—like livestock farming, which didn't require the strength necessary for the heavy plow, making it a job that was equally favorable to men and women alike. Shepherdesses and milkmaids rapidly expanded in numbers, mainly employed in return for money, room, and board. A usual condition of their employment was that they had to remain unmarried and without child—the appearance of a husband or a baby was grounds for dismissal. That helped push up marriage ages, which reduced birth rates. In turn, in a Malthusian economy, that helped keep wages high.[57]

But while the northwestern corner of Europe enjoyed growing freedom for the peasantry, across the Mediterranean and in Eastern Europe peasants were forced to perform *more* labor for their lord, losing rights to move and the right of access to royal courts. The different outcome was in part because it was easier for peasants to run off to a town in comparatively urbanized Western Europe than it was in the east, and also because grain prices didn't collapse in the east as they did in the west, thanks in part to government grain monopolies.[58] That considerably weakened the bargaining position of agricultural laborers—and the serf system remained in place into the nineteenth century. In a step back to the times of Justinian, Venice even imported slaves from the Caucasus to help farm in Crete.

The Black Death continued scarring Europe for far longer than had the plague of Justinian. The Great Mortality was followed eleven years later by the Children's Plague. That killed off as much as a fifth of the English population, focusing especially on those born since the Black Death itself (many older people had immunity from surviving the initial wave). And epidemics struck again and again—fourteen times in the Netherlands before 1500.

The good news, such as it was: plagues became both more localized and less deadly, with mortality rates that merely struck down one in every ten of those living instead of up to one-half.[59] Perhaps better building standards played a role. Europeans were increasingly living in structures made of brick, stone, and beams rather than wattle and daub. Perhaps the displacement of *Rattus rattus* (the comparatively companionable plague rat) by *Rattus norvegicus* (which is more wary of humans) helped reduce the likelihood of infection.

• • •

And what of William McNeill's theory that plague ravaged China before coming west? Historian George Sussman argued that "we still cannot state with any degree of assurance whether the Black Death . . . even visited China or the Indian subcontinent in the fourteenth century." He notes there are no firsthand descriptions of plague or its symptoms in Mongol sources or from Silk Road travelers anywhere to the east of the Caucasus in the entire century.[60] The plague first appears in Indian texts in the early seventeenth century, when the Mughal emperor Jahangir himself reported that "it became known from men of great age and from old histories that this disease had never shown itself in this country [before]." And while China's population halved over the course of the thirteenth and fourteenth century, and epidemics undoubtedly played a role in that alongside war and natural disasters, the first description of a Black Death–like plague in China is from a local gazetteer from Lu-an, Shanxi, in 1644.

In 2010, a genetic analysis of plague samples from disinterred victims appeared to support McNeill's view of a source in or near China.[61] But more recent exercises involving a greater number of samples have pointed to central Asia as the potential source, closer to modern Kyrgyzstan, which would fit with Sussman's view of where it likely began.[62]

Why was the south and east of Asia likely saved from the Black Death? In the case of India, Sussman suggests distance, the geographical barriers of mountains and deserts, and maybe fewer of the right kind of rat and flea. For China, one factor may have been the nature of the trade along the silk road: we've seen that, as in ancient times, Europe ran a trade deficit with the East: slaves from central Asia and silks, porcelain, and spices from China went one way, much of what went back the other was silver and gold. That might suggest rats, fleas, and disease had an easier time going west than east. Another factor might be that Chinese cities were comparatively clean and spread out, which lowered pest populations.

Economists Voigtländer and Voth argue that the plague played an important role in the relative fortunes of China and Europe over the next few hundred years.[63] In the century of the Black Death, China was the font of global technological progress, unified and governed by a career bureaucracy chosen by competitive exam. And yet as the plague was petering out in the eighteenth century, still well before the age of coal and steam, England's average income and the proportion of the population living in cities in Western Europe as a whole were both twice that of China. How to explain it?

Voigtländer and Voth suggest that the reason for the reversal in economic fortunes between China and Western Europe was the Malthusian system at work: the plague increased incomes more in the West than in the East because it was more devastating in the West than in the East. The impact of the plague may be one major reason that Europe became the source of colonizers and conquistadors two centuries later.

In the other direction, the Black Death eventually reached Iceland and perhaps even Viking settlements on Greenland. Given the contact between those settlements and Vineland on the coast of North America, the New World had a lucky escape—it was not exposed to the plague of the fourteenth century. The peoples of the Americas were not so lucky a century and a half later, when explorers from Europe rediscovered the continent with far more devastating effect.[64]

CHAPTER FOUR

Pestilence Conquers

Great was the stench of the dead. After our fathers and grandfathers succumbed, half of the people fled to the fields. The dogs and vultures devoured the bodies.

—*The Annals of the Cakchiquels*

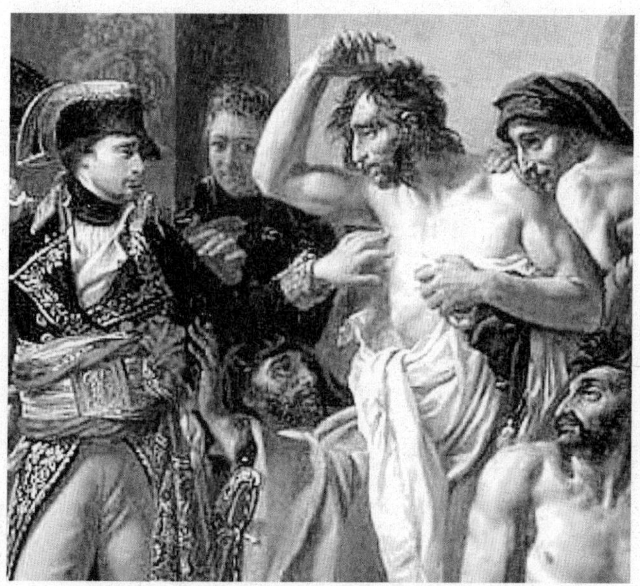

Napoleon, who suffered multiple defeats thanks to infectious disease, sticks his finger in a bubo. The detail is from Antoine-Jean Gros's painting *Napoleon Bonaparte Visiting the Plague-Stricken at Jaffa.*

(Source: *Bonaparte Visiting the Victims of the Plague at Jaffa*, March 11, 1799. Baron Antoine-Jean Gros, 1804. Wikimedia Commons)

Around twenty thousand years ago, people lived on a large land bridge between Siberia and Alaska that submerged at the end of the ice age. As the glaciers retreated, the survivors were able to expand into the Americas even as they were cut off from Eurasia. Within two thousand years they'd spread across rich hunting grounds from modern Canada to the ends of South America.[1]

A number of the larger native mammals became extinct soon after, a process potentially sped up by hunting, climate change, and diseases brought by humans themselves. That may have been one reason to adopt farming, but by that point there were few species left to domesticate—guinea pigs, turkeys, ducks, llamas, and alpacas.[2] As it happens, these animals are host to few microbes that can easily jump to humans. Isolated from most Eurasian diseases of civilization, and incubating few new diseases of their own, the first Americans suffered largely from the microbes of prehistory—including herpes viruses, anthrax, worms, and (possibly) yaws, which is related to syphilis.[3] Hence, ensuing millennia saw steady population growth. The number of humans may have been suppressed by trying to farm without horses, oxen, cows, and pigs, but the scarcity of fellow-traveling bacteria and viruses conferred a net health benefit.

By the 1480s, as described in Charles Mann's *1491: New Revela-*

tions of the Americas Before Columbus, both North and South America had developed civilizations with considerable cities and empires. Varied estimates suggest the continents held between 40 and 80 million people (that compares to Europe with 74 to 88 million).[4] The civilizations of the New World built pyramids, carved stepped roads through mountainsides, developed complex calendars, and fashioned beautiful artwork out of metals.[5] And in 1491, the Inca controlled the world's largest empire—bigger than Ming dynasty China.[6] The conurbation of Tenochtitlán, Texcoco, and Tlatelolco in Mexica was much larger than Paris and its surrounding suburbs—Europe's largest metropolis at the time.[7] But in a matter of decades, these civilizations were overrun by Eurasian and African microbial invaders.

In the years after the Black Death, the Mongol Empire fragmented. The rising Ottoman Empire spread from Anatolia through the Balkans and down to the Indian Ocean. It took its own toll (literally) on trade from the Far East to the West. And European adventurers became increasingly enamored of the idea of another route—a way to reach the silks and spices of the East by sea. Compare the horse or camel and its carrying capacity to that of even a rather modest ship; it's clear that sending goods on a distant journey via the ocean would take less time and require less effort and negotiation than to emulate Marco Polo and try to cross the steppe.

Christopher Columbus treasured his manuscript copy of Marco Polo's *Travels*, and it helped fire him to his own adventures.[8] While Portuguese explorers planned routes around Africa to reach the Indian Ocean, Columbus imagined a more direct route—straight across the Atlantic to Cathay. On his first voyage, he found neither China nor spices, nor significant quantities of gold. Instead, he carried back iron pyrite—fool's gold—along with bark that wasn't cinnamon and chilies that weren't pepper.[9]

Columbus also found people, noting they were "very well built with fine bodies and handsome faces . . . fairly tall on the whole, with fine limbs and good proportions." Ominously, he also reported "they have no iron. . . . All the inhabitants could be taken away to Castile or held as slaves on the island, for with fifty men we could subjugate them all and make them do whatever we wish."[10] He told his royal sponsors that with another trip across the Atlantic he could manage so much more: "To speak only of the results of this very hasty voyage, their highnesses can see that I will give them as much gold as they require . . . also I will give them all the spices and cotton they want."

Though Columbus was unable to deliver on his promise after his second voyage, the Americas would provide all of this and more in time.[11] But the cost that the peoples of the New World would pay for the explorer's ambitions was foretold by his first return trip: of the seven enslaved Americans that Columbus brought back with him to Spain to prove his discoveries and provide translation on the next expedition, only two survived the voyage.

When Europeans, including Columbus, first described Native Americans, they praised them as healthy and strong, while American Indians told one another that Europeans were small, weak, smelly, and diseased. This last point was accurate and deadly—because the interlopers passed on those diseases to their unwilling hosts. Meanwhile, the Spanish conquistadors who trekked across the New World didn't suffer from greatly increased disease mortality themselves—the Americas didn't host a range of new killer infections that they hadn't been exposed to before. A Spanish settler, who arrived on Hispaniola in 1502, looked back eighteen years later at what had become of the island as a result. Hernando Gorjon reported that many Spaniards had left, while "the pestilence of smallpox, measles, flu and other illness they had given to the Indians" had killed off most of the natives.[12]

The death toll of European discovery mounted as the Spanish moved to the mainland. When Cortés, conquistador and secretary to the Spanish governor, first reached the Yucatan at the start of the sixteenth century, there were still as many as 16 to 25 million people in central Mexico. In 1519, he led twelve hundred Spanish troops into the Aztec capital Tenochtitlán, where he was welcomed by Emperor Montezuma. Cortés briefly imprisoned the king in the palace of Lord Face of Water—and the king was soon dead. Montezuma's brother Cuitláhuac was quick to revenge the former king, and Cortés was lucky to escape with half his force over a temporary bridge in the dead of night. But Cuitláhuac didn't press his advantage—perhaps because he was already dealing with the hideous impact of infections that were surging on the mainland within months of Cortés arriving. Some diseases may have hitched a ride aboard one of the first Spanish slaving vessels to travel from Africa to the New World.[13]

And so when Cortés tried conquest a second time with the support of local allies two years later, his most important weapon had already been deployed: infection was savaging his opponents, killing as much as one-half the population—including Cuitláhuac in 1520.[14] *The Annals of the Cakchiquels*, records of Mayan people living in what is today's Guatemala, report that "great was the stench of the dead. . . . Half of the people fled to the fields. The dogs and vultures devoured the bodies."[15] When Cortés and his army reached Tenochtitlán, they overcame the remaining opposition—although enough survived that Cortés was able to slaughter as many as forty thousand within a day of his arrival. There were so many dead, the explorer boasted, "we were forced to walk upon them."[16]

As Cortés's triumph suggests, disease was considerably abetted by the immense violence of the new colonists. Bartolomé de Las

Casas arrived in the New World only ten years after Columbus had discovered it. In 1502, at the age of eighteen, he became a land and slave owner on the island of Hispaniola. Eight years later, he was ordained a priest, but in that same year he was denied confession by Dominican friars on the grounds he was a slaveholder. It took four years, but the Dominicans' message eventually had an impact: in 1514 Las Casas accepted that massacring and enslaving the local population might not be a terribly Christian approach, and he spent much of the rest of his life campaigning for their better treatment. In 1542, he wrote his *Short Account of the Destruction of the Indes*, which described the invaders' "unjust, cruel, bloody, and tyrannical" warfare. "It is the Spaniards' custom in their wars to allow only young boys and females to live," he complained, and added a description of oppression of those who remained: "the hardest, harshest, and most heinous bondage to which men or beasts might ever be bound into."[17] By 1620–25, after repeated bouts of diseases, including smallpox, plague, and measles, exacerbated by violence and maltreatment, the population of central Mexico had collapsed.

European diseases spread faster than European explorers did. That meant, by the time conquistadors and colonists arrived, local civilizations across North and South America were weakened or falling apart already.[18] After infecting the Aztecs, for example, European diseases raged their way south, traveling the roads of the Inca Empire. Smallpox reached the capital of Cuzco by 1524, where it killed the royal family and thousands of warriors. That plunged the civilization into a desperate civil war exploited by Francisco Pizarro, who captured the Inca Emperor Atahualpa in 1532.

In 1541, Pizarro's half brother Gonzalo led an expedition into the Amazon in search of the legendary city of El Dorado. While he failed to find the city of gold, his second in command, Francisco de Orellana, did become the first European to navigate the Amazon.

A Dominican chaplain accompanying Orellana reported that "the farther we went the more thickly populated" was the land around the river, with villages less than a crossbow-shot apart and numerous large cities. It appears that, before 1492, areas fifty miles wide or more around the Amazon and its major tributaries may have been densely occupied all the way into Peru and the base of the Andes, twenty-five hundred miles from the sea.[19]

The scale of infectious destruction along the Amazon was so massive that disease in the Americas achieved what the Black Death had failed to do in Europe: complete social breakdown. The few survivors were reduced to a Stone Age forest existence, their descendants to be found today among "uncontacted tribes" like the Yanomamo. The idea that development is always arrested by tropical climates is simply not true in the case of the Amazon basin. It was *reversed* in part through the introduction of Old World diseases that thrived in such climates.[20]

And the reversal wasn't limited to South and Central America: agriculture occurred in as much as two-thirds of the territory of the United States before Columbus, argues Charles Mann. The scattered tribes that were met by Lewis and Clark during their exploration of the Louisiana Purchase were remnants of a massive farming culture destroyed by disease.

For many of the colonizers, the disease advantage was a sign of heavenly favor. Pilgrims and missionaries suggested the intervention of "the good hand of God" in the smallpox epidemics killing off Native Americans—a case of the Almighty demonstrating that he "wishes that they yield their place to new peoples."[21] This nod of approval by Providence justified exploitation, and the Spanish colonizers relied on native populations for cheap slave labor—even though directly enslaving them was eventually banned by the Spanish king.

As native populations collapsed under the weight of infection, colonists had no choice but to look elsewhere for people to mine the metals and harvest the tobacco and sugarcane. In parts of the New World, a second option was indentured servants: Europeans contractually obliged to work for plantation masters until they'd paid off the cost of their transatlantic voyage. About three-quarters of Virginia's settlers in the seventeenth century, along with the majority of Caribbean field labor until the middle of that century, were indentured.

From the earliest days of colonization, African slaves were brought in alongside servants to meet the demand for labor. Slavers would often advertise that their merchandise displayed the scars carried by smallpox survivors, which meant they were immune to re-infection. Nonetheless, slaves brought with them a range of tropical diseases. These were deadly not only to Native Americans, but also colonists.

By the late 1600s, the more lethal form of malaria, falciparum, had been introduced from Africa to the Americas along with yellow fever—a condition that rendered men prostrate with headache and muscle pain before they'd heave black vomit, endure convulsive deliria, and fall into coma and death. Colonist death rates climbed, and new indentured servants became harder to find. Demand for slaves further increased.

Those slaves who survived the "Middle Passage" across the Atlantic were treated worse than livestock. Anyone who attempted to flee was burned alive or left to rot in a gibbet.[22] Beatings, rape, and malnutrition were the lot of those who stayed. In Haiti, a slave in Saint-Domingue described the conditions: "Have they not hung up men with heads down, drowned them in sacks, crucified them on planks, buried them alive, crushed them in mortars? Have they not forced them to eat shit?"[23]

But despite the obscene conditions in which they were kept, slaves were less likely to succumb to falciparum than Europeans or native Americans because they'd been "seasoned" by exposure and some were more genetically resistant to the disease due to the sickle cell trait. The mortality rate for British soldiers of European descent in Jamaica was more than three times higher than that for soldiers of African descent in the colonial period—and malaria plays a significant part in that differential.[24] The greater hardiness of slaves from malarial regions was soon plain to see, and these captive workers began collecting particularly high prices at auction—as much as 60 percent higher.

Elena Esposito of the University of Bologna has uncovered a simple correlation: across countries, the higher colonists' mortality, the higher the population of slaves. Again, within the US, the greater the risk of falciparum malaria across US counties, the greater the importation of slaves.[25] As late as 1860, moving from an area where the risk of falciparum malaria was very low to one where it was very high was associated with an increase of more than one-quarter in the ratio of slaves in the total population, Esposito suggests.

Farther north, where climate was unfriendly to tropical disease, Europeans remained, if anything, healthier than they'd been in the fetid villages and towns of the Old World. And because they were more seasoned to infections that thrive in cold weather, like influenza, whooping cough, and measles, they were also better adapted to the emerging disease ecology than African slaves.[26] Between 1620 and 1642, only about one in twenty English people arriving in the Caribbean and North America landed in New England. But they survived and thrived in newly depopulated territories rather than falling to disease.

A century after Cortés had triumphed with the vital aid of smallpox, the Pilgrim Fathers were to benefit to a similar extent: an epidemic almost annihilated the Massachusett people of the Algonquin nation only a year or two before the Mayflower arrived.[27] With plenty of sparsely populated, pre-cleared, easily occupied land to take from the poxed Algonquin, the pilgrims rapidly multiplied. Parson Malthus was inspired to write his tract on population in part by the explosive growth of the North American colonies that, he estimated, doubled in size every twenty-five years.[28] Had he grasped all of the factors behind that growth, he might better have understood the role of disease as a check on population.[29]

Ultimately, in both North and South America, Old World peoples and their diseases almost completely displaced local populations. By the year 2000, some parts of the "New World" were made up of populations entirely from the Old, including Jamaica and Haiti. In many more—including the US, Canada, Cuba, Argentina, and Brazil—the descendants of the New World were less than 10 percent of the population. Only in a handful of countries in the Americas are Old World descendants the minority.[30]

The demand for labor created by collapsing populations in the Americas would have a dramatic impact on the unwilling source for that labor. In fact, the slave trade would prove to be the powerful first blow of European imperialism against Africa, wiping out civilizations there.

The Portuguese captain Diogo Cão explored the mouth of the Congo River and met with representatives of the Kongo kingdom in 1482. By 1526, King Afonso of the Kongo was reduced to writing begging letters to the king of Portugal over the behavior of slavers in his country:

> Merchants are taking every day our natives, sons of the land and the sons of our noblemen and vassals and our relatives, because the thieves and men of bad conscience . . . grab them and get them to be sold; and so great, Sir, is the corruption and licentiousness that our country is being completely depopulated.[31]

The Kongo king's appeal for controls over the slave trade went ignored—indeed, the trade rapidly expanded. Between the fifteenth and nineteenth centuries, 12 million slaves were exported from Africa—around twice the population of the United Kingdom in the seventeenth century, although still less than the number of Native Americans that died from the conquistadors' army of disease.[32]

The eventual result was the collapse of the Kongo kingdom and others. Slaving set not just kingdom against kingdom but village against village, each vying to capture enough slaves to sell in return for weapons for self-protection and to take yet more slaves in the future. The slave merchants supplying labor to a New World denuded of people by infection couldn't have created a better mechanism to spread Hobbesian disorder had they tried.

And the slave trade itself spread infection, perhaps eventually killing off more than those who embarked on slave ships. Prior to the era of European exploration and slaving, trade routes had crisscrossed Africa for centuries. But the routes operated on a relay system—goods would be transported by the local population to the edge of its area of control, then passed on to porters from the next ethnic group. The approach may have evolved as a disease-avoidance technique.[33] Certainly it limited contact and kept Africa a continent of many disease pools.

The relay approach obviously couldn't work with slavery—moving people was the very essence of the trade. As a result, smallpox spread throughout Africa. Falciparum malaria may have expanded its reach by the same route. Some estimates suggest the population in Africa by the mid-nineteenth century was half what it would have been absent the impact of the slave trade.

Economists, including Daron Acemoglu and James Robinson, authors of the bestselling analysis *Why Nations Fail*, suggest that colonial disease burdens can explain a considerable amount of variation between rich and poor countries today. That is because places where colonists rapidly succumbed to disease (including Central America and the Caribbean) were left with institutions that favored a small elite raking off incomes as rapidly as possible before retreating from the disease threat.[34] These institutions survived decolonization and fostered inequalities that have festered. Meanwhile, Harvard economist Nathan Nunn shows that "the African countries that are the poorest today are the ones from which the most slaves were taken."[35]

Similarly, research by Stelios Michalopoulos and Elias Papaioannou of the Center for Economic Policy Research suggests that areas of Africa controlled by powerful centralized states before colonization are richer today.[36] Their measure of regional wealth is how much light is visible from space at night—areas with more street lighting and houses spilling light out of their windows are better off than areas where the roads are unlit and homes are dark. It turns out this is a good indicator of average incomes in a region. Areas ruled by stronger states hundreds of years ago are brighter at night today. Given the slave trades' terrible impact on precolonial African states, visiting aliens might not even need to land on the planet to witness some of the legacy of slaving and the infectious diseases that spurred its growth.[37]

• • •

The Age of Discovery was the beginning of the age of truly worldwide pandemic threats. Venereal syphilis provides an early example: it may well have been a New World disease brought back to Europe by sailors from Columbus's original expedition.[38] In its initial foray in Europe, it was far more virulent than it has become, causing ulcers, tumors, immense pain, and frequent death.[39] As a sign of the increasing integration of the global disease pool, syphilis reached the Middle East by 1499 and China ten years after that.[40] India was hit dramatically quickly—in 1498.[41] That is because five years after Columbus reached America, Vasco da Gama became the first European of modern times to round Africa's Cape of Good Hope, and he did it with a syphilitic crew.

As the sailing ships of Europe circled the globe, island after island suffered similar consequences from an explosion of infections. The final great discovery of the age of exploration occurred in 1769, when James Cook landed in Australia and started the last great continental kill-off of unexposed populations. Where North America was repopulated with slaves and indentured servants, Australia started off with British convicts. The difference was of little significance to the Aborigines. Like the native peoples left in North America, they ended up at the bottom of the pile—overwhelmingly disadvantaged in terms of income, education, and health to this day.

Owing in part to an almost complete travel and trading ban with the rest of the world that had been in place from the 1630s, Japan held out against the full global microbial apocalypse for another ninety years. The lower disease burden was an important factor supporting one of the densest populations in the world. The city of Edo had a population of about 1 million in the early eighteenth century, considerably larger than the population of London at the time.[42] But in 1853, US commodore Matthew Perry led four ships into Tokyo Bay, and returning the next year with a larger squadron, he signed the Treaty of Kanagawa with a grudging Japanese government: the country would open two ports for refueling and provisioning American ships. Disease followed soon after, including epidemic typhus and bubonic plague.[43]

But it wasn't a one-way relationship from globalization to infection. Just as disease set the limit to urban growth, it also limited imperial growth. That's because, from the earliest empires, armies campaigning far from home were particularly susceptible to disease—both local microbes as well as the infections that always haunted large masses of people congregated together without adequate sanitation.

For the vast majority of history it was this infection, far more than wounds suffered in battle, that killed off the most troops. To quote the Harvard biologist Hans Zinsser from his entertaining and path-breaking study of the impact of infectious disease on history written in 1935:

> In point of fact, the tricks of marching and of shooting and the game called strategy constitute only a part—the minor, although picturesquely appealing part—of the tragedy of war. They are only the terminal operations engaged in by those remnants of the armies which have survived the camp epidemics.[44]

The wise men of the ancient world were well aware of the risk of unsanitary camp conditions. Deuteronomy (23:12–14) reports that Moses was fastidious when it came to keeping camps clean, for example: "Thou shalt have a place also without the camp, whither thou shalt go forth abroad: And thou shalt have a paddle upon thy weapon; and it shall be, when thou wilt ease thyself abroad, thou shalt dig therewith, and shalt turn back and cover that which cometh from thee."

But concern with camp cleanliness wasn't enough to stop huge numbers of troops throughout history from dying of infection. For example, three different crusades were stymied by three different illnesses: plague, dysentery, and typhoid. Between 1098 and 1099, a Christian army that took Antioch and Jerusalem was reduced from three hundred thousand to sixty thousand men, largely by infection. And nearly all of the half-million-strong army of the Second Crusade perished in a similar manner.[45]

It wasn't just—or even mostly—the troops: one example of the carnage wrought by the microscopic camp followers of far less deadly armies is Europe's Thirty Years' War in the seventeenth century, sparked by religious conflict in Germany. In France, mortality rates may have as much as doubled, and the Holy Roman Empire itself lost 5 to 6 million people—more than a third of its population.

Along with plague, typhus is one of history's biggest killers. It emerged in epidemic form at the end of the fifteenth century, and rapidly became a particularly effective (if indiscriminate) weapon of military destruction in conflicts including the Thirty Years' War. Typhus is spread by lice, including *Pediculus humanus corporis*—also known as the cootie or clothing louse. As an infected louse feeds on its host, it defecates bacteria-laden feces, and when the victim scratches their itching bite, that action rubs the feces into the wound.

As bad as this is for the host, it's no picnic for the louse either, as the sympathetic Hans Zinsser relates:

> If lice can dread, the nightmare of their lives is the fear of some day inhabiting an infected rat or human being. For the host may survive; but the ill-starred louse that sticks his haustellum

> through an infected skin, and imbibes the loathsome virus with his nourishment, is doomed beyond succor. In eight days he sickens. In ten days he is *in extremis*, on the eleventh or twelfth his tiny body turns red with blood extravasated from his bowel, and he gives up his little ghost.[46]

Typhus bacteria breed in the lining of small blood vessels. The infected cells slough off, block the vessels, and stop the flow of blood—starving surrounding tissues of nutrition and oxygen and breaking the vessels open. The condition begins with chills, fever, headache, and a rash, followed by back pain, coughing, insomnia, and—in terminal cases—delirium, coma, and death. In the Thirty Years' War, typhus was spread by desperate, dirty, and ravaging armies short of food—ones even more than usually despising of local populations on the wrong side of the religious divide.[47]

The threat of disease was also one reason why European colonization in the tropics, in particular, was so limited until the nineteenth century. In 1805, Scottish explorer Mungo Park led an expedition to Timbuktu (in modern Mali), and all but two of his forty-strong team of European expeditionaries died of infectious diseases. That was a far from unusual outcome. Death rates for British troops stationed at home in the 1820s were around fifteen for every thousand troops. In India, they were twice to five times as high. In the West Indies, they were six to nine times as high and in West Africa, thirty-two to forty-five times as high. Around half of those stationed in West Africa died *each year*—nearly all from disease.[48] The risk of death was only worth it if there was potential for massive returns (in the case of the sugar industry), or limited contact (in the case of the slave trade from Africa). It simply wasn't possible to set up large, centrally managed colonies across most of the tropics because soldiers would die too quickly to retain control.

Emperor Napoleon was perhaps the last great imperialist to see world-spanning ambition dashed by the microbe. He successfully imposed his rule (or satellite status) on Spain, Switzerland, the Italian states, Prussia, Sweden, and Austria, and extended the borders of France as far as Denmark in the north and through the Italian Piedmont in the south. But his ambitions spread even farther—Napoleon had dreamed of an empire stretching from the bayous of Louisiana to the steppes of the Russian plain and the upper reaches of the Nile. At all three geographic extremities, disease destroyed his armies. In 1798, General Napoleon invaded Egypt and Syria. The adventure was not his finest military hour. Plague killed thousands of his troops and helped end a campaign already marred by poor planning and lack of equipment. Egypt was returned to the Ottomans with the support of the British army in 1801.

In the same year, Napoleon sent his brother-in-law, Victor-Emmanuel, along with twenty thousand troops to Haiti to depose Toussaint Louverture, a former slave who'd risen up against imperial rule a few years before. The emperor wanted to use Haiti as a base for the creation of a Mississippi Valley colony. General Victor-Emmanuel Leclerc won some resounding early victories, but between January and April of 1802 he lost his own life, the lives of the considerable majority of his original troops, and more than thirty thousand reinforcements to yellow fever.[49] By 1803, the battle for Haiti had been lost. Napoleon abandoned his American colonies and sold the territory of Louisiana to the United States for the bargain price of $15 million.

For another decade, Napoleon had considerably more luck in Europe. By 1812, the empire and its dependencies stretched from Spanish Algeciras to Warsaw. But his campaign against Russia in that year was thwarted in large part by typhus. Of the half million or so troops that had crossed the Nieman River into Polish Russia in June, perhaps twenty thousand re-crossed it in December.

By the time of the Napoleonic Wars, typhus was a well-known threat. As the emperor marched through Poland, his army surgeons warned him that the local population was rife with the illness. Napoleon ordered no contact between his soldiers and Polish people. But the army's supply train was foundering behind, along roads ill-designed for heavy wagons. The orders were ignored as troops went in search of something to eat.[50]

Jakob Walter, a stonemason, had been drafted into Napoleon's army. He later wrote an autobiography in which he reported his experiences in the Russian campaign. He suggests that troops were already hungry enough to be slicing meat off live pigs and eating it raw as they reached the Russian border. Three days into Russia, marching through a swamp that provided nothing in the way of forage or fuel, Walter "lay in the tent shelter cold, hungry and wet." He was thankful soon enough that comrades "who came in and lay down upon me served as warm cover."[51] So, no doubt, were the lice that accompanied them.

The emperor's surgeon general, Dr. Dominique-Jean Larrey, reported that sixty thousand men were judged sick by their commanding officers, and the true figure was probably twice as high.[52] Dysentery, hepatitis, and a host of other conditions played a role, but it was typhus that was expanding to epidemic proportions. By mid-August—only two months into the campaign—the French army's effective fighting force was only a little more than a third its size in June, and that attrition had occurred before there'd been a single major military engagement.[53]

On September 7, at Borodino, the French and Russian armies finally met. By the end of that day, writes Stephan Talty in his history of the campaign *The Illustrious Dead*:

> The French had lost 28,000 men . . . the Russians, about 45,000, roughly half of their entire frontline troops. . . . It was the deadliest engagement in the annals of warfare to that date. It would take a hundred years, until the battle of the Somme, for the totals to be exceeded.

But while the Russians retreated in the end, Napoleon failed to destroy their army, or dent the Russians' commitment to the war. Typhus had taken from Napoleon the troops he'd needed for decisive advantage, argues Talty "and with them the battle, the war, and the future of the empire."[54]

Imagine the scenes in the army hospitals of the French after Borodino: Surgeon General Larrey himself performed two hundred amputations in the day after the battle, rarely pausing to wipe off instruments between each cut, or even each patient. Wounds to the chest or stomach were usually considered simply too dangerous to operate on. Patients were left to recover—or more likely die—where they were. For those disemboweled by cannon shot, the mess of intestines was cleaned off as best as possible, stuffed back into the body, and covered with a linen bandage. The room would have stunk with the fecal matter of those who'd lost their digestive tracts and those who'd merely lost control of them—that along with the fetid smell of gangrene. The air would have been filled with screams of un-anaesthetized victims losing a limb to a surgeon's blunt saw, its teeth likely still clogged with the cartilage and bone of the last patient. And around the walls, delirious typhus victims in the last stages of the disease would have added to the din. As those sufferers died, an army of lice, carrying the disease with them, would have found new hosts—dooming many of those lucky enough to avoid serious infection from wounds or the surgeon's saw.

Napoleon marched onward to Moscow. Foot soldier Jakob Walter reports that there were beets and cabbage aplenty to be foraged around the city, as well as a break in the cold weather, but neither lasted long.[55] The army camped with no sign of Russian surrender. After weeks more of losses to disease, malnutrition, and encroaching starvation, the emperor ordered retreat, abandoning thousands of the sick to the mercies of the returning Russian government. At the start of the long march back to Germany, he was reduced to seventy-five thousand troops, less than one-sixth the force he'd had at the start of the campaign.

As the army made its way through poor agricultural lands already stripped of what had been available on the march in, as the temperatures dropped, and as Russian troops harried the retreating columns day after day, the situation became increasingly desperate for all but the parasites. Walter writes that "the fighting, the shrieking, the firing of large and small guns, hunger and thirst, and all conceivable torments increased the never-ending confusion. Indeed even the lice seemed to seek supremacy, for their number on both officers and privates was in the thousands."[56] At the request of his major, Walter tried to kill the lice in the officer's shirt collar, "but when I had his collar open, his raw flesh showed forth where the greedy beasts had gnawed in. I had to turn my eyes away with abhorrence." Recognizing that his own body was similarly infested, he tried to comfort himself with the aphorism that "lice stay on healthy people only."[57]

Vilnius, the capital of Lithuania, was toward the end of the retreat. Only twenty-five thousand troops reached the town. And only three thousand were to leave it. In August 2001, construction workers in Vilnius were tearing down an old Soviet army barracks. As they cleared the foundations, the workers came across a mass grave—seven corpses in each square meter of ground over an area almost twenty meters a side—two or three thousand bodies in all.

The corpses were still dressed in fragments of uniform from the French Imperial Army. Examining the bodies, researchers from the University of the Mediterranean in Marseilles looked for evidence of what had killed them. The scientists found that fully one-third had been infected by louse-borne diseases.[58]

Walter reports that as he traveled back home through Wurttemberg as one of the few survivors "we were shunned like lepers" and locked in a house together. It did not matter—as many as 250,000 died in Germany from the typhus brought back from Poland and the Pripet Marshes.[59] Walter himself recovered from a fevered illness thanks, he suggests, to a course of vinegar and bleeding. Invalided out of the army, he lived at least until 1856—a very lucky exception to the vast majority of Napoleon's invading force. Napoleon himself fought on for three more desperate years until his final defeat at the battle of Waterloo, his dreams of global empire ultimately reduced to Longwood House on the prison island of St. Helena in the South Atlantic.

If civilization created a firestorm of disease, disease also set the limits to the scale of urbanization. And if globalization merged disease pools, the pools crucially shaped the nature and extent of colonization and commerce. Throughout most of history, humanity's only major effective response to infection—exclusion—helped ensure those limits remained. Only with the sanitation revolution was urbanization and integration freed from the constraints of infection, and only with vaccination and antibiotics did that process go global.

CHAPTER FIVE

The Exclusion Instinct

> Reports of illegal immigrants carrying deadly diseases such as swine flu, dengue fever, Ebola virus, and tuberculosis are particularly concerning.
>
> —US Representative Phil Gingrey, 2014

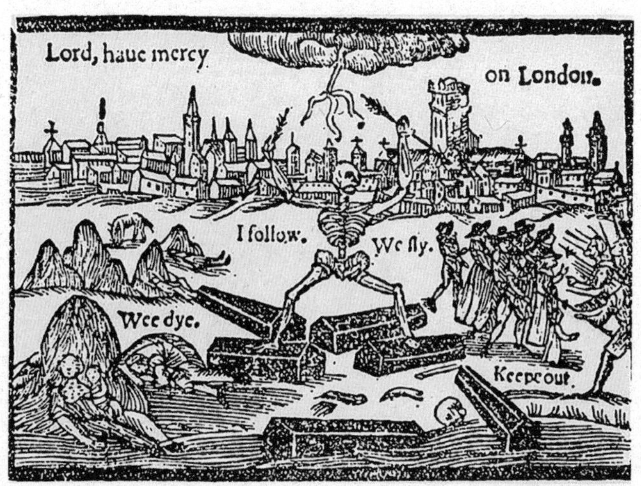

Plague victims fleeing London are told to "Keepe out" by locals. (Credit: H. W. Haggard, *Devils, Drugs and Doctors*. Wellcome Collection. Attribution 4.0 International [CC BY 4.0])

When it comes to evolution, the survival of the fittest applies as much to the risk of being killed from *within* as from *without*. And this has had an impact on both biology and behavior. Humans have inherited and evolved biological defense mechanisms to counter microbes, but they've also evolved behavioral responses, including a preference for cleanliness and a distaste for the diseased. Exclusion and sanitation both build on those behavioral traits.

To begin with the biological defenses, sex may be one early response to infection. If you budded from your mother, you'd be her identical twin and susceptible in exactly the same way to exactly the same infections as she was. Sex mixes up genes—some of which might help defend against particular diseases. That makes it less likely one parasite can wipe out a whole population.[1] (And in the case of Covid-19, the sex of the infected person may make a difference to mortality rates, with men dying more frequently than women among early cases.)

Another evolutionary response to disease is the white blood cell. AIDS—acquired immunodeficiency syndrome—gives us an idea about what life would be like absent those infection-fighting cells, because the disease destroys them. AIDS sufferers experience very low white-blood-cell counts, and rapidly acquire a range of infections as a result. Pneumonia and tuberculosis (the blood-coughing lung disease) are frequent AIDS fellow travelers. The HIV virus that causes AIDS uses our defense mechanisms against us: one evolved response against infection (sex) to attack another (the white blood cell).

As a cause of most human deaths over thousands of years, infection has also fostered genetic diversity among the world's human populations. This diversity isn't by any means the primary factor in whether a person dies from an infectious disease or survives it. The rate of evolution of rapidly reproducing viruses and bacteria is distinctly quicker than the rate of human evolution, suggesting the lethality of various infectious diseases probably has a lot more to do with their evolution than with ours. That's one reason it's so difficult to know what diseases people are describing in the distant past: they've often evolved since then. But people whose ancestors lived many centuries in areas that were hospitable to particular diseases have sometimes inherited somewhat more effective biological responses to those diseases.[2]

Take malaria: it's caused by a tiny protozoa, a single-celled organism. Carried by the mosquito and injected with the saliva that the insect uses to prevent clotting as it sucks blood, the parasite travels through the bloodstream to the liver, where it grows and multiplies. Eventually the malaria organisms burst out of the liver cells that have nourished them and re-enter the bloodstream, invading red blood cells, feeding and multiplying again, before destroying cells in a coordinated attack and floating onward to infect another—or to be sucked up into the gut of a mosquito feeding on the prostrate body of the malaria victim.

As the millions of red blood cells collapse, the human host shivers even as their temperature shoots up. The host suffers blinding headaches. If they're lucky, the fever breaks in a few hours—at least until the next round of blood cells collapses under the onslaught. If the host is *unlucky*, enough infected blood cells crowd the brain to block the transfer of oxygen. The person becomes unconscious, enduring muscle spasms that weaken as he or she slips toward death.

Malaria used to be present in countries as far north as the UK.[3] But there are different variants of the protozoa, some more lethal than others. And falciparum malaria, the most deadly variant, is concentrated in Africa between the Sahara and South Africa. Some people in that region developed a costly genetic defense against the disease—the sickle cell trait. Red blood cells in people who inherit the trait from one parent form a distinctive sickle shape when oxygen is limited, and that apparently helps them resist the malaria parasite. But in people who inherit the genetic trait from both parents, blood cells constantly form in the sickle shape, which can lead to anemia, and increases the risk of stroke, organ damage, infection, and heart failure.

It's a sign of the health risk of malaria in tropical Africa that this dangerous genetic condition has lasted, simply because it can be a partial defense against the disease. The genetic marker for sickle cells is present in nearly one in five people in northern Angola and around one in ten in much of the rest of the continent south of the Sahara and north of South Africa. Outside of Africa, the sickle cell trait is very rare because, historically, its costs considerably outweighed benefits in areas with less lethal malaria strains, meaning people with the trait were more likely to die, so less likely to have children and pass on that trait to the next generation.[4]

Another example of an inherited effective biological response is the human leukocyte antigen, which is associated with recognizing microbes within the body. Justin Cook of the University of California-Merced has found that those in or descended from European and Middle Eastern regions have high levels of human leukocyte antigen diversity. Africans come next, and the original native populations of the Americas and Oceanic states last (both because of less evolutionary pressure connected to disease but also because the original inhabitants were a smaller group of humans in the first place).[5]

But it's worth emphasizing again that genetic variance hasn't made any group immune from a disease that affects the rest of humanity—doubtless in part because diseases have evolved in response. And the limits to the biological protections against disease help explain why animals, including humans, have developed a whole range of different instinctive responses to reduce their exposure to microbes.

Any time a horse stamps its hoof, tosses its head, or twitches its tail to disperse flies, it's demonstrating an instinctual response to infection. Many animals go to great lengths to avoid fouling their nests with their own feces, while others, including baboons, rotate roosting sites so that any individual site is clear of parasitic larvae by the time they return. Sheep and cattle all avoid eating forage that is close to recently dropped feces or (in the case of cattle) areas laced with tick larvae.

Disgust is a human instinctual response to infection risk according to scientists at the London School of Hygiene and Tropical Medicine. There are, they suggest, "a universal set of disgust cues . . . including bodily wastes, body contents, sick, deformed, dead or unhygienic people, some sexual behavior, dirty environments, certain foods—especially if spoiled or unfamiliar—and certain animals."[6] Worldwide, contact with these cues leads to shuddering, grimacing, heightened blood pressure, reports of nausea, and the desire to withdraw. The relationship between infectious disease risks and these universal disgust cues is clear.

Disgust is also a source for fears of contact, and especially sexual contact. This is probably why the idea of barriers to the flow of body fluids as a disease preventative is very old indeed. The first mention of a condom-like device to stop the transmission of a deadly condition appears in Greek mythology, when King Minos of Crete used the bladder of a goat over his penis to protect his wife Pasiphae from the serpents and scorpions that swam in his semen and would routinely kill those with whom he had intercourse. Apparently, neither the scorpions nor the goat-bladder condom prevented Minos from fathering more than a dozen children. (The couple were well matched: Pasiphae's tryst with a bull while disguised in a cow costume led to the birth of the Minotaur.)

Disgust cues may also lie behind beliefs linking bad smells to sickness—the "miasma theory." Vegetius's *de Re Militari* (in English: *Concerning Military Matters*) is a fourth-century CE text on the training, logistics, strategy, and tactics of the Roman Army. Among other things, it's the source of the maxim often repeated by military industrialists: "Let him who desires peace prepare for war." But the book also contains advice on sanitation that displays miasma thinking at work: "If a large group stays too long during the summer or autumn in one place, the water becomes corrupt, and because of the corruption, drinking is unhealthy, the air corrupt, and so malignant disease arises which cannot be checked except by frequent changes of camp."[7]

Fear of disease is also, of course, a source of the instinctual fear of strangers. When newcomers attempt to join a troop of primates, they're kept at the outskirts of the group and often threatened by dominant group members for weeks or months before being admitted. While this may also involve protection of food resources or the exclusion of breeding rivals, one reason for the behavior may be to expose infection and allow it to run its course before a new member is fully admitted. Think of it as a primate form of quarantine.[8]

Staying away from infected people and keeping infected people away is a reasonable strategy. Continent-level isolation is what kept the original Americas and Australia free of so many Old World infections until the last few hundred years. At a local level, quarantine and social distancing can reduce the average number of new people each person with the disease goes on to infect. In some cases (and the less contagious the disease, the easier this is), limiting connections between people in an infected community can drop the number of new people each disease carrier infects to below one. If you manage that for long enough, the outbreak dies out.

The 2003 SARS coronavirus outbreak, in which infected people rapidly showed clear symptoms, was controlled through quarantine measures. Cross-country tracing and isolation of people who'd been in contact with a known SARS victim quickly found and sequestered the majority of all the people who were infected by the virus worldwide.[9] Even if it's hard to completely end a large-scale outbreak of a more contagious, less obvious disease in the same way as SARS, you can at least slow its spread by keeping people apart. That is why isolation and social distancing were both introduced in 2020 to reduce the chance that Covid-19 sneezed or coughed out by an infected person reached a previously uninfected host.

The instinctually understood reality that isolation can be effective may be one reason why surveys from around the world in the spring of 2020 found considerable majorities in favor of lockdown and social distancing strategies—more than 70 percent in Senegal and about three-quarters of Americans in mid-April, for example.[10] It may also be why when you make study participants think about infectious disease—showing them pictures of someone with measles, perhaps—those participants report themselves less keen to socialize with others than people who haven't been shown the pictures (and so probably aren't thinking about disease).[11] Worryingly, test subjects made to think about infection also show more racial prejudice.

And this experiment encapsulates the checkered history of exclusion through the ages: a sometimes reasonable response to disease threats evolves all too frequently into a mindless justification for deadly prejudice. Nativists, racists, bigots, and the rich have always been prone to use disease outbreaks combined with the exclusion instinct as an opportunity to act on their theories of superiority. Often left unsaid but nevertheless implied is that a disease has flared up because of the moral or intellectual failings of the victims, their genetic inferiority, or their lack of manners.[12]

The earliest written sources suggest that people have long appreciated the risk of contagion and understood the benefits of exclusion. For thousands of years cities have confined disease sufferers to their quarters, and in the earliest civilizations, officials sometimes obligated soldiers returning from campaigns to burn their clothing and shields.[13]

An association between disease and exclusion has also shaped a number of religious customs. The Book of Leviticus in the Bible includes detailed instructions for diagnosing, isolating, and treating victims of leprosy (not the condition we now know of as Hansen's disease, but another ailment):

> When a man shall have in the skin of his flesh a rising, a scab, or bright spot, and it be in the skin of his flesh *like* the plague of leprosy; then he shall be brought unto Aaron the priest . . . and the priest shall look on him, and pronounce him unclean. . . . And the leper in whom the plague *is,* his clothes shall be rent, and his head bare, and he shall put a covering upon his upper lip, and

> shall cry, Unclean, unclean. All the days wherein the plague *shall be* in him he shall be defiled; he *is* unclean: he shall dwell alone; without the camp *shall* his habitation *be*. . . . And on the eighth day he shall take two he lambs without blemish. . . . And he shall slay the lamb in the place where he shall kill the sin offering and the burnt offering, in the holy place.

Treatments also involve the sacrifice of turtle doves, alongside the plentiful use of cedar wood, fine flour, and oil.

Because of the natural fear of contagion, ministering to the infected has long been associated with devotion and morality, and that's particularly true of the condition that came to be called leprosy in the Middle Ages: Hansen's disease itself. An apocryphal story tells of the future King David I of Scotland in 1100 coming upon his sister, wife of King Henry I of England, who was kissing the feet of lepers with devotion. David warns that her husband will never kiss her again. His sister replies, "Who does not know that the feet of an Eternal king are to be preferred to the lips of a mortal king."[14]

Compare that with Diana, Princess of Wales, nine hundred years later, suggesting, "It has always been my concern to touch people with leprosy, trying to show in a simple action that they are not reviled, nor are we repulsed."[15]

The infected suffer lesions that can damage facial bones and the extremities as well as nerve endings, all to the point that fingers, toes, and even whole limbs may fall off. Hansen's disease is not in fact very contagious: only communicable after prolonged exposure and (apparently) only to the hereditarily predisposed. Lifelong quarantine is an unnecessary and cruel response. But the Chinese Book of Han in 2 CE reports that leprosy victims were sent to a hospital where they were isolated.[16] Similarly in Europe, in the first

250 years of the second millennium, the misapplied biblical suggestion of uncleanliness made those accused of leprosy subject to religious dictate over treatment.

Once pronounced leprous after priestly or magisterial examination, the victim was taken under a black cloth to the altar, where a priest threw earth from the cemetery over his or her head, uttering "dead unto the World but alive unto Christ." The priest read out a list of prohibitions against entering churches, taverns, or marketplaces, talking to someone upwind of their body, traversing narrow lanes, or touching wells, streams, fountains, or children. And then the leper was led out of town to the lazar house, where they would live with fellow sufferers. The leper's property was passed on to inheritors, and the only legal recognition of his or her continuing earthly presence was that a wife couldn't divorce an infected husband.[17]

Nineteen thousand leprosarium or lazar houses operated across Europe, stationed on the downwind side of towns. They were filled with victims of Hansen's disease and others who a priest, magistrate, or jury had determined were at least deserving of the condition.[18] The moral nature of leprosy was made clear by Richard of the Abbey of St. Victor in Paris in the 1200s: "Fornicators, concubines, the incestuous, adulterers, the avaricious, usurers, false witnesses, perjurers, those likewise who look upon a woman lustfully . . . all are judged to be leprous by the priests," he wrote.[19] Confession was thought the only cure, lechery the likely cause.

Along with Jewish people, lepers were ordered to wear special clothes by the Catholic Church in 1215, and the occupants of lazar houses were regularly accused of the same plots and conspiracies, and suffered the same horrible consequences. In 1321, King Philip V of France became convinced that the heads of lazar houses were planning to poison wells with reptile parts and human excrement in an attempt to contaminate all of France with leprosy. Under torture, some lazar heads admitted the plot, and claimed funding had come from Jews and distant Muslim kings. Across France, lepers were tortured and burned at the stake—inevitably, Jewish people were burned alongside them. Not for the first or last time, disease victims weren't only blamed for their condition but mistrusted and maltreated as a result.

In 1364, Guy de Chauliac, Pope Clement VI's doctor, listed the marks and signs of leprosy in his manuscript *La Grande Chirurgie*. The list became a standard reference tool used by doctors when they were called to provide evidence at leper trials, and helped end the mass incarceration of those accused of incubating the condition.[20] As we'll see, de Chauliac wasn't as successful when it came to responding to the Black Death—the great health disaster of his age—but he did report one theory about the plague's origin: "In some places, they believed that the Jews had poisoned the world." It was a conspiracy theory that was to have grim consequences, because alongside the hideous natural death toll, others died at the hands of those looking for a "foreign" scapegoat for the disease.

On April 13, 1348, the year the Black Death returned to Europe after an eight-century absence, the Jewish quarter of Toulon was sacked and forty victims were dragged from their homes and murdered. In the following days, surrounding towns and villages followed suit. These were the first of a series of brutal attacks across Europe as rumors spread that the plague was the result of Jews poisoning wells under the instruction of a rabbi named Jacob, who was set on world domination. By the end of 1348, the popular madness surrounding well poisoning had spread throughout much of Germany. The Jewish population of Basel and Strasbourg were herded into specially constructed houses that were set on fire. In Speyer and Worms, Jewish communities headed off murder through mass self-immolation. More than two-thirds of the German towns with significant Jewish populations saw pogroms between 1348 and 1350.[21] We've seen that anti-Semitism was not created by the plague, but the plague gave anti-Semites a murderous excuse. (And the roots ran deep: people in areas where more plague-related pogroms occurred in the fourteenth century were considerably more likely to vote for the Nazi Party in the 1930s, a half-millennium later.)[22]

Jews were the most horribly treated but not the only suspect group to be singled out as exclusion became the public policy response to the plague. Over time, health commissioners began regulating schools, church services, religious processions, and the movement of beggars, soldiers, and prostitutes. Authorities could lock people into their own houses, seize and burn belongings of the sick, or send victims to pest houses. (Death rates in those houses soared thanks not just to plague but malnutrition, starvation, and other infections of the abandoned.)[23]

Argues historian of medicine Dorothy Porter, health legislation "was targeted at restricting the movements of the morally outcast, such as prostitutes and sodomites, 'ruffians' and beggars, as well as the plague sick-poor, who were assumed to pose equally serious threats to civil order."[24] As with leprosy, the plague was considered a judgment on the unworthy.

Eugenia Tognotti of the University of Sassari notes that medicine "was impotent against plague; the only way to escape infection was to avoid contact with infected persons and contaminated objects."[25] So social distancing made sense. The Florentine writer Boccaccio, who reported on the failure of his city's efforts to keep the plague away, describes one strategy to survive in his fictional account of a group of men and women who abandon the plagued city altogether and retreat to an estate two miles out of town. He suggests those who thought "there was no medicine for the disease superior or equal in efficacy to flight" were "the most sound, perhaps, in judgment, as they were also the most harsh in temper."[26]

And sufficient isolation really worked: in a later plague outbreak in France from 1720 to 1722, nearly nine out of ten villages with fewer than one hundred people were spared a case of the plague altogether. Compare that to mortality that reached 30 to 40 percent in large towns.[27] Staying away from urban concentrations of rats, fleas, and people—in cut-off, largely self-sufficient farming communities—was a smart move.

But commentators at the time wondered if some of the exclusionary measures did more harm than good—and they had a point. There's good reason to doubt that isolation in houses slowed the movement of rats that helped carry plague, and significant grounds for thinking isolation and incarceration of the sick along with healthy relatives did harm.

The regulations certainly increased the power of health officials. And because disinfection and quarantine were expensive—cleaning out 1,536 homes in Milan in 1576 cost the equivalent of more than one hundred pounds of gold—taxes rose rapidly in cities undergoing a plague epidemic.[28] Alongside war, public health became a major force behind the growing scale of government.

Another health-safeguarding idea that gained currency was restricting the arrival of peaceful people from other cities and states, since plagues always seemed to come from "elsewhere." Florence imposed fines on visitors from plague-affected cities and appointed a municipal health commission with the authority to forcibly remove infected persons (the stated reason was that "a corruption or infection of the air" might arise from them).[29]

In 1348, Venice kept ships in the harbor from docking for thirty days to see if those on board came down with the plague. Venetian colonies followed suit. In Marseilles in 1383, the isolation period was extended to forty days, and as that practice spread, it came to be referred to as "quarantine" (*quaranta* is the Italian for "forty").[30]

The proliferation of sea and land quarantines may have helped reduce the extent of later plague pandemics. Four thousand troops manned the southern border in Austria-Hungary, holding many travelers in quarantine for as long as forty-eight days, fumigating trade goods, and putting suspect goods in a warehouse. People were considered expendable enough that if they developed plague symptoms, they could be shot. The last major plague outbreak in Western Europe, in 1720, was traced to a ship that had evaded the quarantine system by bribing the authorities. It went on to kill one hundred thousand people in and around Marseilles.[31]

The association of disease with outsiders—either socially undesirable or geographically distant—continued through the centuries. Take syphilis, first recorded in Europe in the armies of Charles VIII of France, fighting in Italy in 1494 (newly returned members of Columbus's crew were among the troops). As that army disbanded, it helped spread the disease across Europe, where it became known variously as the Naples Disease, the Spanish Sickness, the French Pox, the German Sickness, and the Polish Sickness, depending on the course of its spread and the traditional national prejudices of the country most recently infected.[32] When it reached the Middle East, it was called "the European Pestilence." And the Japanese labeled it "the Chinese Pox." (Similarly, the Irish were blamed for bringing cholera to the US in 1832, the Italians for spreading polio, and tuberculosis was called "the Jewish disease.")

Syphilis's clear association with sex made it a convenient weapon of those trying to outlaw prostitution. Many fifteenth-century towns had, alongside sanctioned town brothels, municipal baths that were home to prostitutes—in London, they were concentrated in Southwark, on lands owned by the bishop of Winchester. But as knowledge of the new disease spread, the attraction of casual sex reduced. The scholar Erasmus, noting the decline of steam baths in Brabant in 1526, reported that "twenty five years ago, nothing was more fashionable. . . . Today there are none, the plague [syphilis] has taught us to avoid them."[33]

A moralizing attitude toward syphilis continued despite widespread understanding that condoms could protect against the disease. The Ancient Egyptians used linen sheaths to prevent sexually transmitted disease, and the Romans followed the Greeks in the use of animal bladders.[34] Gabriele Fallopio, an Italian anatomist who lived in the first half of the sixteenth century and gave his name to fallopian tubes, described his invention of a made-to-measure sheath of linen soaked in salt water tied with a ribbon at its base. He also claims that he gave eleven hundred men sheaths to use during sex and not a single one caught syphilis when using one of them.[35] Mrs. Perkins, purveyor of "implements of safety," who advertised her condoms for "ambassadors, foreigners, gentlemen and captains of ships," did more for public health and, in particular, women's health in eighteenth-century Britain than people like Malthus who suggested abstinence was the only acceptable way to avoid either pregnancy or disease—but Malthus was long on the winning side.

Alarmed by the proportion of army recruits rejected on the grounds that they were syphilitic, Britain introduced the Contagious Disease Acts in the middle of the nineteenth century, which forced prostitutes in garrison towns to register. Those identified as "common prostitutes" by the police were subject to physical inspection using the (incredibly unsanitary and invasive) steel penis of the speculum. Women declared diseased were locked up in quarantine hospitals. (Men, it should be noted, weren't subject to inspection or punishment.) As late as the First World War, the British rejected issuing condoms to troops, on the grounds that soldiers were better sick than enticed into mortal sin (again, nothing was said about the effect on women).[36]

A greater understanding of the biology of infection increased pressures for the use of exclusion to preserve public health. The germ theory of disease became scientifically dominant thanks in large part to the work of the Frenchman Louis Pasteur and the German Robert Koch in the second half of the nineteenth century.

In 1876, Koch extracted anthrax bacteria cells from a diseased animal, grew the bacteria in his lab, and then transmitted them to healthy animals to give them the disease. Over the next eight years he followed that up with discovering the organisms responsible for tuberculosis (previously thought to be inherited) and cholera (a favorite of those who thought stench caused disease). Koch used his newfound status to call for extended quarantines and isolation. Many of Koch's initial dissenters were motivated to oppose the germ theory in part by fear of what it implied for public policy. Take Florence Nightingale, nurse-hero of the Crimean War:

> "The disease-germ fetish, and the witchcraft-fetish, are the produce of the same mental condition. . . . The germ hypothesis, if logically followed out, must stop all human intercourse whatever, on pain or risk of disease or death."[37]

Nightingale's fears were prophetic. Isolation remains a powerful tool to reduce the spread of disease, but when it is applied as a permanent measure to "high risk groups" rather than sick individuals, exclusion can be the cause of considerable harm.

By 1889, homeowners and medical attendants in the UK had the duty to report a range of diseases—from smallpox and diphtheria through measles and whooping cough. Medical officers could then decide whether those affected should be isolated at home or in a hospital and whether to disinfect homes, clothing, and bed linen.[38] At the turn of the century, tuberculosis victims in Britain and elsewhere were frequently locked up in sanatoriums, segregated by sex, and subject to strict discipline.[39] The British public "was becoming acclimatized to a new medical rationality which might involve the trimming of its liberties," suggests historian of medicine Dorothy Porter.[40]

Exclusion was a particularly big problem when germs were used as an excuse to keep out and maltreat whole ethnic groups with no more scientific basis than the theory that Jews poisoned wells to start the Black Death. The US Immigration Act of 1891, which provided a foundation for federal oversight of migration, banned criminals, polygamists, prostitutes, contract laborers, and those with a "loathsome or contagious disease." Poor immigrants and those from outside of Europe faced harsher medical scrutiny—thick necks were taken as a sign of goiter, shortness of breath as a result of lung diseases, rashes as evidence of ringworm. In 1898, only 2 percent of all those denied entry into the US were excluded on medical grounds, but by 1915, the percentage had climbed above two-thirds.

Similarly, US officials on the Mexican border oversaw a process whereby migrants were stripped, showered with kerosene, examined for lice, and vaccinated against smallpox. Some of the first undocumented immigrants into the US were those who, in the 1910s, crossed unwatched sections of the Rio Grande rather than submit to invasive medical examination and disinfection.[41]

The third recorded plague pandemic also involved a racist response to infectious threat. It emerged in Yunnan, China, in the 1850s and spread via Canton to Hong Kong, where, in 1894, Alexandre Yersin identified the bacteria that caused it (it was named *Yersinia pestis* in his honor). From there, the steamers of the British Empire took the lead in transporting it worldwide.

Plague arrived in San Francisco in 1900. Echoing a conflict that had raged since the very first quarantine in Dubrovnik and continues today, business interests lined up against government officials in charge of health over the question of imposing movement restrictions.[42] But it's hardly as if those calling for quarantine were acting under the most rational (or noble) assumptions, as was demonstrated when the quarantine was finally imposed. It was applied solely to Chinatown and anyone of Chinese descent trying to leave California.

On May 19, 1900, San Francisco medical staff swarmed over Chinatown restraining anyone who looked Chinese and attempting to inoculate them with an experimental plague vaccine. Chinese merchant Wong Wai brought a suit against the San Francisco Board of Health, claiming that compulsory inoculation was "a purely arbitrary, unreasonable, unwarranted, wrongful and oppressive interference" with his liberty. The judge, William Morrow, agreed on the basis that the compulsory order had been "boldly directed against the Asiatic or Mongolian race as a class, without regard to the previous condition, habits, exposure or disease, or residence of the individual." As such, it clearly violated the right to equal protection under the law guaranteed by the US Constitution.[43]

The ingrained response to keep distance from a person suspected of being sick continues to this day. During the AIDS epidemic, Delta airlines tried to ban HIV-positive people from flights, and Tulsa authorities drained a swimming pool after a gay group used it. (Meanwhile, US senator Jesse Helms called for a reduction in spending on AIDS care because "deliberate, disgusting and revolting conduct" had caused infection in the first place.)[44] From 1990 to 1993, HIV-positive Haitian immigrants were held at Guantánamo Bay, one of many instances to come of America's using the island to ignore human rights standards that would be required on its own soil.[45] And it wasn't just the US—many countries worldwide imposed some sort of restriction on the entry or stay of foreigners with HIV.

Or consider Ebola: the disease is featured in a number of movies because it kills so horribly, leaving victims a bleeding sack of infection. In 2014, West Africa suffered history's worst Ebola epidemic. The outbreak killed thousands before Ebola disappeared back to its animal reservoir, thanks in part to curfews, isolation of sick people, and safe burial of disease victims. But complicating the response, local people in infected areas became markedly unfriendly to medical staff trying to help them. Doctors and nurses arriving to collect victims were threatened with machetes and stones, and their cars were surrounded by angry mobs telling them to leave. In July, staff from Doctors Without Borders, a Western NGO, told the *New York Times* that it "is very unusual that we are not trusted" and complained that people were turning for help to local witch doctors instead of foreign NGOs.[46]

On September 16, 2014, an official delegation reached the village of Womey in southeast Guinea to spread news about the Ebola threat. They also sprayed bleach and water on cars and common areas as a preventative measure. As the aroma of oxidant spread through the compound, the rumor started that the officials were spraying the Ebola virus itself. Village women began to chant "What do you do when someone comes to kill you?" The men replied: "We will kill them." The delegation's security guard fired a warning shot and chaos ensued. Two days later, police found eight bodies of delegation members in a latrine ditch, many with their throats slit.[47]

Meanwhile, halfway around the world, Georgia representative Phil Gingrey wrote to the US Centers for Disease Control and Prevention noting "reports of illegal immigrants carrying deadly diseases such as swine flu, dengue fever, Ebola virus, and tuberculosis are particularly concerning."[48] The reports might have been more concerning had they turned out to be true, but they show that people all over the planet still respond with broad exclusionary instincts to infectious disease risk.

In the past few years, the risk of leprosy, tuberculosis, and even bedbugs has been used by US television and radio pundits as justification for turning back travelers and immigrants.[49] Sadly, Covid-19 provoked similar responses, with reports of increased abuse of Asian-Americans in the United States and Europe, and of worsening discrimination against Africans in China. Particularly monstrous was the stabbing by a Texan of a two-year-old and a six-year-old because he thought they were Chinese and spreading the disease. Xenophobia clings to many official responses as well, including recent travel bans.

Our instinctual response toward disease threats may even have shaped the nature of whole societies. The "parasite stress" theory of attitudes and behavior suggests that the more infectious diseases are present in an area, the more people are afraid of strangers, keep to their own communities, and show violence toward others. Across countries, those with historically higher infectious disease prevalence have populations that are less individualistic, more willing to respect authority, and less likely to want people of a different race as neighbors. They're also more conformist and willing to restrict rights and liberties, according to Mark Schaller and Damien Murray of the University of British Columbia.[50]

Though there is an intuitive appeal to a relationship theory in which disease breeds distrust which breeds conservatism, the evidence mustered to date by parasite stress theorists is more circumstantial than beyond reasonable doubt.[51] It would be a considerable mistake to fall into a state of "pathogen determinism."[52] Schaller and Murray themselves are careful to point out that culture can change rapidly. But pathogen stress—an ingrained behavioral response to a high disease burden—may still be one factor in shaping societies, potentially with long-term consequences. More positively, the theory also suggests that a world of declining disease threats should be one of greater peace, liberty, and cohesion, with lower pressures toward exclusion. That would be good news, because, though historical and modern evidence suggests that isolation and social distancing can be effective in slowing the spread of infection, these measures frequently fail in the long run—and even where they do work, they often carry a high cost by trapping the healthy along with the sick and disrupting trade and travel.

However necessary, Covid-19 exclusion has tragically illustrated the measure's immense cost as a response to disease in the modern world; it has spurred the most rapid contraction of the global economy in a century. We'll see that it has also demonstrated the counterproductive futility of most travel bans on a globally connected planet.

Our deepest habitual reaction to disease is one of the most problematic in the aftermath of civilization and globalization. It took sanitation and a medical revolution to push back infection in an age of urbanization and connected disease pools. And it will take public health and further medical advances to overcome Covid-19 and the threats that come after.

CHAPTER SIX

Cleaning Up

All smell is, if it be intense, immediate and acute disease.

—Edwin Chadwick

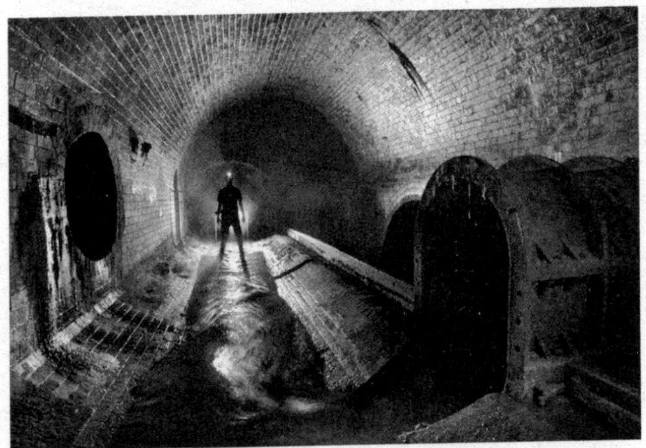

One of Bazalgette's sewers, still operating in London
(Credit: "The Other Aye" by sub-urban.com is licensed under CC BY-ND 4.0)

Like exclusion, keeping clean is a prehuman response to disease threats. Rats spend as much as one-third of their time awake attending to their toilette routines of chewing and licking fur and skin. Primates—apes, not least—spend many hours combing the hair of their fellow pack-mates and picking or even biting off ticks and other bugs. (The high-status apes get the most attention. It isn't just among humans that the upper classes get the best healthcare.)

Cooking is a sanitary response developed by early humans—it kills microbes before we eat them. And, in part, cooking habits might vary around the world thanks to the risk of infection. Paul Sherman at Cornell University and his student Jennifer Billing looked at forty-five hundred recipes for preparing meat from cookbooks across thirty-six countries and found that the hotter the country, the spicier the average recipe. Danish and Norwegian food tends to be bland, Mexican and Indonesian dishes can be blistering. Within China, the (climatically hotter) south prepares hotter dishes than the (climatically cooler) north.[1] Indian dishes use an average of nine spices to England's two.

Sherman and Billing suggest one reason for the link between the heat of the air and the heat of the food: many spices kill bacteria. Garlic, onion, allspice, and oregano inhibit or destroy every bacterium they've been tested on. Spices have to be grown and prepared; that effort is more worthwhile in places where infection from spoiled meat is more likely—hot climates that tend to be "pathogen rich."[2]

But civilization posed an obvious challenge beyond what to load on the spice rack: namely, tens of thousands of people living and excreting in close proximity. More than five thousand years ago, the city of Mohenjo Daro in modern-day Pakistan developed a solution: it boasted many houses with bathing rooms alongside toilets that emptied into covered sewers large enough for a person to walk down.[3] This may have been the global high point for sanitation up until the late eighteenth century, although some ancient Chinese cities constructed similar wonders of hydraulic engineering.

Around 200 BCE, Chang'an, the capital of the Han Empire, relied on an urban water system that included supply, storage, rainwater management, and drainage. Marco Polo's description of Chang'an from a millennium later suggests the city had a huge river on one side and a lake on the other. The "river, which enters by many channels, diffuses throughout the city, carries away all its filth and then flows into the lake, from which it flows out toward the ocean. This makes the air very wholesome." Polo observed that "these people are used to taking cold baths all the time. . . . It is their custom to wash every day, and they will not sit down to a meal without first washing." There were three thousand public baths in the city to clean them.[4]

Chinese cities were conscientious about removing excrement, carting out "night soil" for fertilizer use. And because of internal peace, towns spread beyond their walls, reducing the problem of overcrowding. There were fewer animals crowded into cities as well: the Chinese diet contained little meat. That meant a lower risk of infections shared with livestock.

Polo also noted that the khan regularly entertained forty thousand at a banquet and that the guests apparently enjoyed a high level of sanitary protection. The waiters, some of the khan's barons, "have their mouths and noses swathed in fine napkins of silk and gold, so that the food and drink are not contaminated by their breath or effluence,"[5] a practice that came back into fashion in 2020.

In Europe, imperial Rome enjoyed some of the same sanitary benefits. Aqueducts delivered more than forty gallons of clean water per person per day to the city in the third century CE—feeding private houses, massive public baths, and more than one thousand fountains. Sewage was less advanced, but the Cloaca Maxima, running from the center of the city to the Tiber River, was linked to smaller tributary sewers throughout Rome. Cesspits were emptied at regular intervals, their contents to be used as manure on the fields. And there were specific government offices responsible for maintaining drains, paving and cleaning streets, preventing foul smells, and overseeing baths, brothels, taverns, and water supplies.[6] This—along with the tribute and migrants of empire—is what allowed the city to grow so large.

But as was said earlier, life expectancy in the city remained low—certainly, below thirty years. One reason was high population density. Most Romans were housed in flimsily constructed apartment buildings, supposedly restricted to a seventy-foot height by Emperor Augustus. That would have made the city, one million strong at its largest, a breeding ground for airborne diseases as well as numerous pests, including lice, fleas, rats, and mosquitoes.

The new religion, Christianity, didn't help.[7] Christian observance was enforced in the Roman Empire by an edict in 350. But early Christianity was a dirty religion, one that militated against humans' natural desire to be clean. St. Jerome, who translated the Bible into Latin, typified the problem. As a hermit, he avoided bathing. And he also objected to women engaging in the practice:

> I wholly disapprove of baths for a virgin of full age. Such a one should blush and feel overcome at the idea of seeing herself undressed. By vigils and fasts she mortifies her body and brings it into subjection. By a cold chastity she seeks to put out the flame of lust and to quench the hot desires of youth. And by a deliberate squalor she makes haste to spoil her natural good looks.[8]

A number of other saints clearly felt the same way: St. Benedict had warned against the risks of baths, St. Agnes took none at all in her thirteen years of life, and Catherine of Siena also followed the same routine.[9] The phrase "Cleanliness is next to Godliness" only emerged in the late eighteenth century.

The problem of urban sanitation waxed and waned with the size of cities. Historian John Kelly notes that in fourteenth-century Europe there were at least five Parisian streets named after excrement (rue Merdiere, for example), as well as the rue du Pipi. As long as a person shouted, "Look out below, look out below, look out below!" first, many European towns were fine with throwing the contents of chamber pots out of the window into the street. And continual warfare kept people densely enclosed behind city walls for safety. That was why, in the fifteenth century, life expectancy was a third lower in European towns than in the countryside (the reverse of China's health pattern at the time).[10]

Official complaint about the state of public sanitation became shriller when plague was linked with bad air. King Edward III wrote to the City of London to rail against "human feces and other obnoxious filth lying about in the streets and lanes, where it was cast from the houses both by day and by night, so that the air of the city was polluted with foul odours to the great peril of citizens during that time of prevailing sickness."[11] By 1385, London had a sergeant of the channels on patrol with city rakers who collected filth from the streets and piled it on dumps by the river, where it was collected by dung boats. Officially, fines were imposed for throwing dung onto the road. But the remaining piles of ordure and the few people fined suggest enforcement was lax.[12]

And as London expanded in the Middle Ages, carting dung through congested streets to urban plots or the countryside became more complex. In 1411, Henry Ivory, a London privy-cleaner, earned sixty-five shillings for digging out and carting away 3,675 gallons of ordure—about seventy bathtubs' worth. Each year, he'd remove about three times that total.[13] But not everyone paid for privy-cleaning services, and urban areas were eventually buried in excrement from human inhabitants, alongside dung from horses, cows, and other animals housed with them.

In response, the power of public officials over sanitation continued to expand: in 1486, Venice had an elected Public Health Commission of three noblemen who inspected wine, fish, meat, and water supplies, monitored sewage, and regulated burials to control the threat of miasma. In 1504, they were given the power to arrest and torture people to ensure ordinances were followed.[14] These ideas spread: England's Cardinal Wolsey and Thomas More, both lord chancellors to Henry VIII, introduced plague orders in the second decade of the 1500s that copied many features of the Italian model.[15] Some cities added more controls: London massacred dogs in 1563, while Edinburgh banned leeks, chives, and onions two years after.[16]

Despite a growing role for the state, London's average life expectancy remained only around twenty-eight years, thanks in part to poor sanitation. The increasing piles of animal and human excrement, rubbish, and corpses would have been a direct affront to the senses and created a disgust instinctively associated with disease. By the 1780s, suggests historian J. N. Hays, "air had become the health issue, the nose was the diagnostic tool, and clean water was the solution to the filthy atmosphere that bred disease."[17] The foundations for a sanitation revolution were in place.

In the early 1800s, one in five of the English people lived in towns with a population of more than five thousand. Less than fifty years later, as the Industrial Revolution took hold, that proportion had risen to one-half. Between 1800 and 1850, Birmingham tripled in size while Manchester and Liverpool more than quadrupled.[18] And, by 1870, London was home to 3 million people.[19]

These packed and dirty cities teemed with infections ancient and modern. For many infected by tuberculosis, a disease thousands of years old, the immune response is rapid and effective. The body creates a holding pen for the organism—the tubercle—which stops further damage. But for others, the barrier doesn't hold, and tuberculosis spreads. If it reaches the lungs, victims suffer consumption—a deathly pallor, with coughing fits of bloody sputum.

Tuberculosis had an apparent penchant for striking the suffering artist—in the three years from 1847 to 1849 alone, consumption carried off Felix Mendelssohn, Emily and Anne Brontë, Edgar Allan Poe, and Frederic Chopin. But the efficacy of people's immune response and their ability to live with the disease appear to be related to a range of factors, including general health, nutrition, and stress.[20] And that meant tuberculosis was most lethal among poor, malnourished people packed into growing slums. In the middle of the nineteenth century, it was killing fifty thousand people in England and Wales each year, with rates that varied by orders of magnitude between wealthy and poor parts of the same city.[21]

A new affliction was cholera. The first cholera pandemic emerged in 1817, spreading rapidly thanks to globalization and poor sanitation. Cholera is a bacterial infection that passes from the end extremity of the digestive system of a host to the start of the digestive system of a new victim, also known as the fecal-oral route. It can do so explosively thanks to cholera's symptoms. If someone swallows enough of the microbe, these symptoms can start within hours of infection. Diarrhea develops into "rice water stools"—milky water that is expelled in volumes as much as five liters a day. As the victim's body rapidly dehydrates, the person suffers muscle cramps, plummeting blood pressure, a slowed heart rate, and coma. Death from renal failure and circulatory collapse can be so rapid that even treatment by antibiotics is ineffective.[22]

The first cholera pandemic spread through India with the help of war. The British general the Marquess of Hastings reported death striking victims in as little as a few hours and that hundreds of troops were dying each day. That is to say nothing of those who were unfortunate to live in the path of the various armies. Not everyone was saddened by the losses—the Calcutta Medical Board, loyal Malthusians to a man, suggested that the consequences of the outbreak "may in the present instance have been beneficial, correcting the influence of an overcrowded population."[23]

By 1820, the outbreak had reached China, the Philippines, and (thanks to a British expeditionary force) the Persian Gulf. Two years later cholera was killing people in Japan. Russia and Egypt both imposed quarantines that may have worked at least in the short term—and the disease retreated for a few years. But it roared back: by 1831, it had reached Britain, and in 1832, it evaded North American quarantines and spread along waterways through Canada and the United States.

Over the course of the nineteenth century through the First World War, India lost as many as 25 million people to the disease.[24] In Europe it was no Black Death—mortality was only in the tens of thousands in major cities, killing off one in twenty or one in ten, not one in three or one in two. Nonetheless, it was a sign that growing globalization could produce threats not just to the newly conquered but the conquerors. And the disease came as a rude shock according to R. S. Bray, author of *Armies of Pestilence*:

> Western Europe had been free of plague for over one hundred years, smallpox was on the retreat and yellow fever was but an infrequent visitor. It was only the lesser races which suffered great epidemics in the opinion of nineteenth-century Western Europe. Cholera came as a very nasty surprise indeed and Europe was in thrall to it. It struck terror into the hearts of a civilization which had thought that the external world was softening towards it.[25]

Cholera spread misery and fear.[26] The overwhelmingly poor victims of the infection focused their wrath on the establishment—in Russia, riots erupted around the idea that the aristocracy was using cholera to kill off workers, while in the UK the rioters were convinced doctors spread the disease to increase the number of cadavers available for dissection.[27] Given that the wealthy shared Malthus's concern with the teeming masses, it wasn't implausible they'd welcome or even enable a disease that would thin populations.

In the 1830s and '40s, William Farr, compiler of abstracts of the Registrar General's Office, used the new UK register of births, deaths, and marriages to confirm that death rates were higher where poor people were packed together. He felt sure that unsanitary conditions lay behind the correlation.[28]

Farr's friend Edwin Chadwick had reason to agree with him. Chadwick was a lawyer and essayist turned social reformer who'd implemented Britain's Poor Law. The legislation herded those desperate enough to ask for relief into locked and sex-segregated poorhouses, where they wore uniforms and were denied alcohol, tobacco, or reading material besides the Bible. Chadwick argued that these unpleasant conditions would ensure only those who really *needed* support, rather than the merely lazy, would apply for relief. It was an attitude toward people that fit with his personality: headstrong, impatient, dogmatic, convinced of his infallibility, and utterly humorless. He demonstrated his attitude toward the majority of his countrymen in a letter attached to a set of deficient cutlery he was returning to a silversmith: "My new experience in household matters has brought so much annoyance from the carelessness of workingmen of every class . . . I intend to make these experiences of the indolence and inattention of workmen the subject of some remarks on popular education."[29]

But Chadwick *did* accept that some of those left destitute were disadvantaged by ill health in increasingly foul industrial towns up and down the country. His poorhouses had surely removed the problem of poverty causing ill health because they provided sustenance and shelter to those people who really needed them. Something else must be driving the spread of ill health that itself caused greater poverty. Chadwick's *Report on the Sanitary Condition of the Labouring Population of Great Britain* noted: "The annual loss of life . . . is greater than the loss from death or wounds in any wars in which the country has been engaged in modern times." He suggested the direct cause was "filth and bad ventilation."[30]

In 1846, Chadwick convinced a parliamentary committee that "all smell is, if it be intense, immediate and acute disease."[31] In response, he promoted what he labeled "the sanitary idea": a national and local bureaucracy to provide for clean water and drainage, paved streets, and proper housing together with the control of "noxious trades" like abattoirs.[32] His first step, backed up by an 1847 law: close the cesspits that were the receptacles of the city's human waste and direct excrement through pipes from backyard privies into storm sewers, taking the smells with them. In a period of just six years, thirty thousand cesspits were dismantled and many of the 2 million Londoners began flushing their waste into sewers that led to the River Thames.[33]

Chadwick's priorities, according to the London *Times*, were "the complete purification of the dwelling house, next of the street and lastly of the river."[34] His report suggested that, eventually, intercepting sewers should be constructed on the banks of the Thames to take waste away from the river to be used as agricultural fertilizer. But the priority was to get smelly ordure away from houses.

Chadwick's solution, if fully implemented, would have carried waterborne bacteria like cholera far from London's inhabitants, breaking the chain of infection. But leaving the river to be dealt with sometime later was a fatal problem: the Thames was the source of much of the city's drinking water. The new sewage system helped ensure that cholera microbes could be piped almost directly from sufferer to new victim. Chadwick's half solution was part responsible for a particularly virulent epidemic of cholera in 1848–49 that killed more than eighteen thousand Londoners.

By 1849, water companies, their customers, and the press were all crying out for a solution to the foul water and stinking river. That was the year that engineer Joseph Bazalgette returned to the capital where he had been born three decades before.

As a twelve-year-old, Joseph had witnessed the first cases of cholera reaching London. He'd left the city to work on land drainage projects in Ireland and railway projects in the north of England. But in the aftermath of the latest cholera epidemic, Bazalgette was appointed assistant surveyor to the London Metropolitan Commission of Sewers. Six years later, he became chief engineer of the newly created Metropolitan Board of Works. And over that time, Bazalgette created a plan for radically overhauling the capital's sewage system with a set of intercepting pipes that would collect the rainwater and ordure from existing sewers and transport it out of London downstream, toward the English coast, where it would be pumped into the river.

Bazalgette, too, was a miasmist. The sewage system he constructed was to complement Chadwick's earlier work. But the plan was expensive, and opposition was considerable from those who thought the scheme an unnecessary luxury or—like Chadwick—a waste of fertilizer. In the meantime, an 1854 epidemic of cholera came and went, with twenty thousand more deaths.

Members of the British Parliament were finally motivated to act in 1858 by the smell that wafted through Parliament's riverside windows during the "Great Stink" of that year. The Thames turned almost solid with the output of the sewers. If intense smell was acute disease, the Great Stink was a direct threat to Britain's ruling elite as they worked.[35] The government passed an act to authorize the intercepting sewage system.

The feats of engineering undertaken by Bazalgette involved six main sewers, with a combined length of 100 miles, and 450 miles of new interceptor sewers that connected existing sewage lines. Bazalgette estimated the project took 318 million bricks and nearly a million cubic yards of concrete.[36] And the whole system had to be constructed with constant gradients that ensured available water flow could flush the pipes clear. Along with mastering the complexity of a system that always had to slope downward, it was necessary to acquire a deep knowledge of rainfall patterns, water supply, and usage by the city's residents. Bazalgette noted that the habits of the population were reflected in sewage flow: "the maximum flow in the more fashionable districts of the West end being two or three hours later than from the East end."[37]

For all its complexity and cost—4.1 million pounds in mid-century money, worth perhaps more than half a billion dollars today—the system worked brilliantly. The city's excrement was piped and pumped downriver, past the intakes for water supply. And London's last cholera epidemic would take place in 1866.

Most of Bazalgette's network of sewers is still in use today. Other cities across Britain, the rest of Europe, and America followed with similar solutions over the next half century, with significant impact on health.

The sanitation revolution wasn't just about build-out of sewage and water systems, it was also and crucially about changing attitudes toward their use. In the 1710s, total soap consumption in England was less than 0.2 ounces a day—allocated to washing not just bodies, but also clothes, utensils, and everything else.[38] Until the 1800s, the young man or woman seeking advice on etiquette would be told of the importance of clean hands, face, and hair—with nothing said of the necessity of cleaning the rest of the body.[39] But, over the course of the nineteenth century, with industrializing Britain in the lead, full-bodied cleanliness became a necessity of polite company.

By 1849, when William Makepeace Thackeray described "the great unwashed," it was clear that cleanliness was an aspirational good. Britain's Baths and Washhouses Act of three years earlier had encouraged local governments across the country to open public baths where the poorest would have to pay no more than two pence for clean water and a towel. (These baths were signs of slow progress: as late as 1914, when most houses still lacked their own bath, attendance at big-city baths once a year or more ranged between a fifth and four-fifths of the citizens.)[40] And in the 1870s, the Housing and Crowding Acts led to a slew of building regulations that reduced overcrowding and enforced access to clean water.[41]

• • •

The extent of the sanitation victory is clear from what goes on in modern-day global cities. Take, for example, Per Se, a restaurant in New York City, located just off the southwest corner of Central Park. Fox News declared the eatery, which serves a combination of New American and French cuisine, one of the three most expensive in the world in 2014.[42] With a trio of Michelin stars and starters that include a "pastrami" of Hudson Valley moulard duck foie gras alongside the inevitable ossetra caviar, the tasting menu cost $325 a diner (drinks not included).[43] But a 2014 inspection by New York City health inspectors revealed that Per Se had no hand-washing facility or soap in the food-prep area. Additionally, the inspectors reported hot and cold items held in improper temperatures. New York City forces restaurants to post their health inspection grades in front of the restaurant—and given its violations, Per Se was awarded a barely passing C grade.[44]

The city's health inspectors are a small part of a massive urban public health and sanitation operation. The New York City Department of Sanitation, founded in 1881, today has nine thousand staff and a $1.4 billion budget—most of which is spent on garbage collection, street cleaning, and "waste export" (a euphemistic phrase for paying other places to take Gotham's trash).[45] To get rid of liquid waste—sewage—the Bureau of Wastewater Treatment manages six thousand miles of sewer pipes linked to fourteen treatment plants that process and discharge 1.4 billion gallons of water a day. The bureau has nineteen hundred staff and a $376 million budget.[46]

The eight million residents of New York generate enough waste to employ eleven thousand people to get rid of it—and that does not account for the office buildings, which are served by private trash companies.

In the US as a whole, there are 2.3 million janitors and building cleaners, as well as 1.4 million maids and housekeeping cleaners, according to the US Bureau of Labor Statistics. What about plumbers, pipefitters, and steamfitters? There are 387,000 of those—many involved in building and fixing bathrooms and kitchens. Add in the soap, cleaning compound, and toilet preparation manufacturing industries that employ another 100,000 people.[47] The broad "cleanliness industry" may keep as many as 4.5 million Americans employed—around 3 percent of the labor force.

The sanitation revolution that led to this considerable powerhouse of the modern economy is all that allows a city like New York, with its mass of population living (literally) on top of one another, to work. In an area of 305 square miles, or 0.0005 percent of global land, it contains a larger population than the world as a whole as recently as 4000 BCE, suggesting the power of civilization and agriculture—when combined with modern health and sanitation—to overcome Malthusian constraints on progress.

Improved sanitation came with costs. We'll see that it was a weapon of empire. It was also a gateway to total war, keeping soldiers healthy enough to fight at unprecedented scale. The trench warfare of World War I should have been the gift of the century to microbes. Millions of soldiers living for years packed together in sodden trenches, coughing, sneezing, and excreting in extremely close proximity, periodically exposing themselves to a whole host of injuries that would allow even the laziest bacteria of putrefaction to get ahead and reproduce. Under such conditions, typhus would normally have been rampant, for example. But at least on the Western Front, times had changed. Only 104 cases of typhus were reported among the Allies during the entire war.[48] (Russia failed to control the disease, however: as many as 3 million soldiers and civilians on the Eastern Front died of typhus during the conflict.)[49]

Hundreds of thousands more soldiers were left healthy enough to be crippled by high explosives and metal-jacketed bullets that tore through soft tissues. That so many survived these wounds can be credited to improvements in hospital care. In the American Civil War, medical officer Middleton Goldsmith first used a treatment process for wounds that involved cutting out all the dead and damaged tissue ("debridement") and then pouring a mixture of bromine and bromide of potassium onto the wound. Of his 308 patients, only eight died. Four years later, British doctor Joseph Lister demonstrated his antiseptic technique for surgery, and the widespread adoption of sterilization meant that hospital mortality rates for gunshot wounds were half the Civil War level by the time of the Spanish-American War in 1898.[50] It was a revolutionary change from the standards of Borodino, one that allowed far more soldiers to recover from injuries to fight again: progress, of a sad and twisted sort.

Combined with other sanitary interventions, clean water and sewage helped upend the rankings of causes of death in rich countries. Infectious diseases accounted for about 50 percent of all deaths in the UK in the 1860s. By 1900, infection was responsible for a little more than 40 percent of deaths in both the United States and the UK. Already, heart disease, cancer, and vascular conditions had taken the top spots in the mortality rankings. The decline continued into the twentieth century to the extent that, even before the invention of most vaccines and antibiotics, the US and Northern European death toll from infection had dramatically fallen.[51]

And by the time sewer engineer Joseph Bazalgette died in 1891, after adding flood defenses, river crossings, and street improvements to his list of gifts to England's capital, urban areas had closed most of the health gap with rural areas.[52] English life expectancy, which had stalled for nearly forty years from 1820 to well past the mid-century mark, at last began to climb. In 1870, it surpassed forty-one years—a level it had previously reached in 1582, when Shakespeare was writing his plays and the much smaller population was mostly rural.[53] Life expectancy reached fifty by the first decade of the twentieth century.[54]

Marcella Alsan and Claudia Goldin, at Stanford and Harvard Universities respectively, studied the rollout of clean water and a modern sewage system across US cities around the turn of the twentieth century. Infant mortality among the white population fell from about 17 percent dying before their first birthday in the 1880s to 9 percent in 1915. Alsan and Goldin used evidence from Boston to point out that water and sewage improvements alone may account for a little less than half of that decline, largely thanks to fewer cases of diarrhea related to water laced with fecal matter.[55]

As Alsan and Goldin's results suggest, Bazalgette and his sanitarian allies cannot take *all* of the credit for overall health improvements. Nutrition played a role, too—children and adults alike ate more and better food because families had more income.[56] But sanitation was a far more influential force. In the 1630s, wealthy English people could certainly afford adequate food but achieved a life expectancy of only thirty-nine years. By the start of the third millennium those same wealthy classes were experiencing an average life expectancy of eighty-one years because of sanitation-diminished exposure to widespread infection.[57]

Improved sanitation helps against many diseases, but it makes the biggest difference with those that are less easily spread between humans—ones that require a vector animal like a mosquito, flea, or rat, or that only pass through bodily fluids. The unequal spread of sanitation worldwide meant that while everyone remained at risk of diseases like measles, smallpox, or the flu, which travel easily and directly to a new victim through the air, the rich and sanitary became comparatively free of the rest.

Take the 15 million deaths of the third global plague pandemic: the vast majority of those deaths were in South and East Asia. Europe lost perhaps seven thousand people and the United States five hundred. One factor explaining the difference: for all Europe and the US were comparatively urbanized and connected, they were also comparatively rich, with better quality housing and sanitary systems—and fewer rats and fleas.[58]

The sanitation gap continues to influence the health gap: in 2000, northern Uganda suffered an outbreak of Ebola. Dr. Matthew Lukwiya ran a missionary hospital in the region and took the lead in fighting the outbreak, alerting authorities in Uganda's capital, Kampala, and caring for patients in the hospital.

Ebola isn't highly infectious—for you to catch it, infected body fluids from a victim have to come into contact with your nose, mouth, genitals, or broken skin. But if you're working in 100-plus Fahrenheit conditions in a gown, gloves, and face mask for hours on end, you might be excused for making the deadly mistake of scratching a mosquito bite or wiping sweat from your eyes before scrubbing down. That's why the people who care for Ebola sufferers are the most likely to catch the disease themselves. Twelve healthcare workers at Lukwiya's hospital died. The doctor was only able to thwart a staff mutiny through a combination of threatening to leave, appealing to their professional spirit, and singing hymns.

Eventually, Lukwiya succumbed himself, catching the disease while caring for an infected nurse. He was buried the same day he died, by a team wearing full protective gear that sprayed bleach over the coffin as it was lowered into the ground while the doctor's wife and children looked on. Thankfully, he was the last to die at the hospital, and Uganda's Ebola outbreak ended in February 2001.[59] Lukwiya had stopped the disease from spreading—and he did so largely using the tools of sanitation and isolation.

Ebola is distinctive in that it kills or clears up quickly and is only infectious when victims show symptoms. As a result, each victim tends to infect only a very few more people with the disease. If people caring for Ebola patients protect themselves using caps, goggles, gloves, and gowns, while using bleach to clean any blood, vomit, or feces that spills, and the victim is kept isolated, the average infection rate drops below one, and the Ebola epidemic burns out. That's why the disease is only a major threat in countries with very weak surveillance and isolation capacities, like Uganda and Liberia.

Contrast Ebola with airborne Covid-19: in the latter case, isolation and social distancing slowed spread, and access to clean water for hand washing was important. But even cities with advanced water and sewer systems, along with armies of workers keeping hospitals, streets, and buildings clean, saw the coronavirus spread.

Or think about measles, which spreads through the air even more efficiently than Covid-19. The average number of new people infected by every measles sufferer can reach eighteen among populations where no one has had the disease. In those cases, improved care, including boosting sanitary conditions, can reduce mortality rates, but there's little chance that it will significantly reduce levels of endemic infection. If it weren't for the fact that measles at its worst is a far less deadly disease than Ebola, it would have wiped out much of humanity long ago.

Nonetheless, in the twenty-first century, there's some likelihood that we'll wipe out measles—thanks to the invention and worldwide spread of the measles vaccine. Hopefully, the same technology will soon reduce Covid-19 to a minor threat. As we'll see in the next chapter, for all that the disciples of Bazalgette have prevented many millions of deaths—especially in the industrialized world—it's the followers of vaccine inventor Edward Jenner who've saved the most lives worldwide.

CHAPTER SEVEN

Salvation by Needle

I shall ask if any solid observations have been made from which it may be justly concluded that, in the countries where the art of medicine is most neglected, the mean duration of man's life is less than in those where it is most cultivated.

—Rousseau

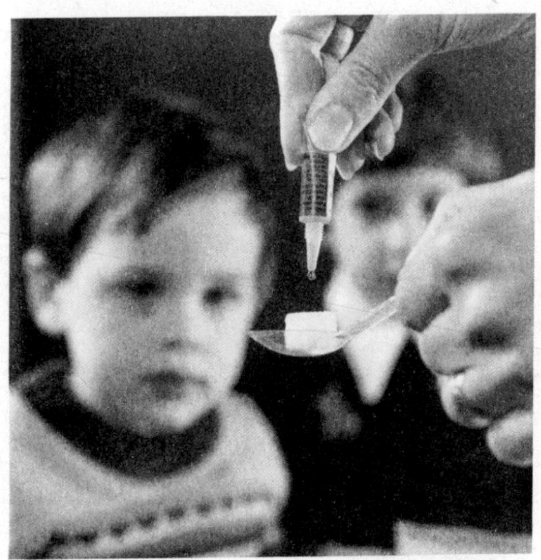

Some vaccines (in this case against polio) can be delivered via sugar cube instead of needle. (Credit: Wellcome polio vaccine. Wellcome Collection. Attribution 4.0 International [CC BY 4.0])

Relying not just on their immune systems and the instincts shaped by the diseases of pre-civilization, civilized humans met the expanded infection challenge with a toolbox that included mostly ineffective treatments (snuff, sacrifice), a short list of more effective sanitary interventions (cooking, clean water), and finally, exclusion of the potentially ill. For most of history, medical advice was often worse than useless in killing microbes or easing symptoms.

Perhaps the greatest doctor in ancient times was Hippocrates, who was born in Cos, in Greece, around 460 BCE.[1] He's nicknamed "the father of Western medicine" in large part because he was firm in the opinion that diseases usually have earthly rather than supernatural causes. Hippocrates was also the first recorded person to suggest the use of an extract of the aspen tree for pain, anticipating modern aspirin.[2]

Hippocrates's ideas regarding the "humors" of phlegm, blood, and black and yellow bile were part of a theory of well-being and illness that dominated much of Western medicine for two millennia. He maintained that human health was determined by the balance of these four bodily fluids. Sickness followed when the humors were out of equilibrium. And bloodletting—cutting open the veins to regain humoral harmony—was a cure.

With halfway bleeding people to death, the state of the art in treatments, it shouldn't be surprising that doctors were often seen as helpless in the face of pandemics. The chronicler of Justinian's plague, Procopius, noted that "the most illustrious physicians predicted that many would die, who unexpectedly escaped entirely from suffering shortly afterwards, and that they declared that many would be saved, who were destined to be carried off almost immediately. . . . No device was discovered by man to save himself." For all the attempts there'd been to find natural causes for disease, Procopius suggested that "it is quite impossible either to express in words or to conceive in thought any explanation, except indeed to refer it to God."[3]

Eight hundred years after Justinian and eighteen hundred after Hippocrates, the poet Petrarch complained bitterly about quackery and punditry during the Black Death: "No remedy is exactly right, and there is no solace. And to the accumulated disaster is added not knowing the causes and origin of the evil. For neither ignorance nor even the plague itself is more hateful than the nonsense and tall tales of certain men, who profess to know everything but in fact know nothing."[4] The advice of doctors regarding preventatives and cures included roasting food rather than boiling it, avoiding milk and meat, and eating lettuce.

Guy de Chauliac, physician to Pope Clement VI who'd described Hansen's disease with such positive effect, survived a bout with the Black Death himself. In 1363, he wrote a medical textbook, *Inventarium seu Collectorium in parte Cyrurgicali Medicine* (*A Partial Inventory of Collection of Surgical Medicine*), that looked back on the first plague outbreaks. "For preservation, there was nothing better than to flee the area before it was infected and to purge oneself with pills of aloe and reduce the blood through phlebectomy," he wrote—retreating to the cure of bloodletting. As for underlying causes, de Chauliac suggested the conjunction of Saturn, Jupiter, and Mars on March 24, 1345, was the major factor, "which made such an impression upon the air and the other elements that, just as a magnet moves iron, so it changed the thick humors into something scorched and venomous."[5]

Not everyone agreed with the leading medical experts of the day. The contemporary chronicler de Mussi noted that the disease spread through ports by way of infected sailors carrying a "contagious pestilence."[6] That cities imposed ordinances designed to reduce the risk of coming into contact with the sick suggests that the possibility that pestilence was contagious was taken seriously. But doctors remained impotent to prevent or cure the condition.

The same was broadly true worldwide. In 1102, China launched a national welfare program that established infirmaries within major cities with the explicit aim of controlling the spread of disease. There were state-sponsored lists of approved medicines, and these were (in theory) often distributed for free at infirmaries. Critics at the time carped at this, and there's no evidence that the system as a whole significantly reduced the impact of such killers as measles, smallpox, flu, and dysentery.[7]

In the West, Vesalius, a sixteenth-century anatomist, used his extensive knowledge of the human form acquired from dissection to challenge the reputation of Galen—the most revered Roman proponent of the theory of humors. Sixty-five years later, William Harvey published *De motu cordis*, which demonstrated the general circulation of the blood. The discovery effectively undermined Galen and Hippocrates's model. In 1637, the French philosopher René Descartes wrote in his *Discourse on Method* of the hopes that such advances offered:

> It is true that the science of medicine, as it now exists, contains few things whose utility is very remarkable: but . . . all at present known in it is almost nothing in comparison of what remains to be discovered; and . . . we could free ourselves from an infinity of maladies of body as well as of mind, and perhaps also even from the debility of age, if we had sufficiently ample knowledge of their causes, and of all the remedies provided for us by nature.[8]

Less than a century after Descartes wrote this, the first effective if dangerous preventative against one of the greatest infectious killers, smallpox, did finally begin to spread from Asia to Europe, thanks in part to (somewhat) scientific experimentation.

The last person to suffer from smallpox (hopefully ever) was Janet Parker, a medical photographer from Birmingham. In 1978, she was working in a lab that held one of the few remaining samples of the disease worldwide. Somehow, it escaped containment. Parker began to feel unwell, experiencing headaches, backache, nausea, and chills as well as terrible dreams. Then large, red, blistering pustules began spreading all over her body: Parker's skin must have felt as if it were on fire. At a point where she was too weak to stand, she was admitted to a hospital; meanwhile, World Health Organization officials rushed to vaccinate anyone who'd been in contact with her—five hundred people.

Parker's condition deteriorated—her eyes scarred to almost complete blindness, and she suffered renal failure and pneumonia. Soon, she stopped responding to people. Professor Henry Bedson, head of the lab where she worked, was so wracked with guilt that he killed himself. And five days later, on September 11, 1978, Janet herself passed away, joining hundreds of millions or more before her who'd also succumbed to the dreaded disease.[9]

Something akin to smallpox was described in Chinese texts more than sixteen hundred years ago. It may have been present in ancient Rome; others suggest it reached the shores of the Mediterranean by the tenth century and Southern Europe by the thirteenth. Genetic evidence points to the potential for an even more recent evolution of the disease, but it was certainly circulating by the 1500s.[10]

It was an equal opportunity killer, striking down rich and poor alike. Consider England's royalty in the seventeenth century: King Charles II survived the pox as a child, but lost two siblings to the disease. Tragedy struck the next generation, too, when Charles II's only descendent died of smallpox in 1660 while the family was exiled in Europe. That left James, Duke of York, Charles II's brother, in the line of succession. He became king in 1685. James's career was nearly as unsuccessful as his father's (who was beheaded at the end of the English Civil War), and he was deposed in the "Glorious Revolution" that put William of Orange and James's daughter Mary on the throne.

But the thirty-two-year-old Mary was herself struck down by smallpox. As Donald Hopkins relates, William, "whose father had died of smallpox the week before he was born, who had lost his mother to smallpox when he was ten years old, and who had had a severe case of smallpox himself as a child, now prepared to bury his young wife, a victim of the same savage illness."[11] William was succeeded by Mary's sister, Anne, whose only son was killed by smallpox in turn, ending the Stuart royal line.

One of the first truly effective preventative treatments against infection had been developed to fight smallpox a century and a half or more before Mary died. Variolation had been practiced in China since at least 1549. The common approach was to blow month-old smallpox scabs up the nose of the patient. (If it wasn't possible to wait a month, the scabs were suspended in steam scented with herbs.) Unbeknown to it's practitioners, this had the effect of killing off or weakening much of the viral material, reducing the risk of a bad case of smallpox.

The Kangxi Emperor, who ruled from 1661 to 1722—during the same time the Stuart line was being erased by smallpox—boasted that he'd inoculated his whole family along with the army, and all had passed through mild cases of the disease. By that time, variolation was also widely used in India. There, the approach was to dip a needle in a smallpox pustule and then stab it in the skin of the patient, which was the approach that ultimately spread west.[12]

Smallpox inoculation as practiced in the Ottoman Empire was written up in the *Philosophical Transactions* of Britain's Royal Society in 1714, which led to an active correspondence. Massachusetts minister Cotton Mather wrote to the society to say that his slave Onesimus, who'd been born in southern Libya, had undergone the procedure. The Turkish version of inoculation involved putting pus from smallpox lesions in the scratched skin of the patient. Usually, that led to a comparatively mild case of the disease because the microbe's preferred transmission route is via the lungs.

In 1715, British aristocrat Lady Mary Wortley Montagu was struck with the pox, but survived—if without eyelashes. In that same year, she traveled to Turkey with her husband, the new ambassador to the Empire of the Ottomans, where she witnessed an inoculation. In one of a stream of amused, charming, and utterly self-confident letters she wrote to friends while abroad, she described the procedure:

> "The small-pox, so fatal, and so general amongst us, is here made entirely harmless by the invention of ingrafting. . . . [An] old woman comes with a nutshell of the matter of the best form of small-pox, and asks which veins you please to have opened. She immediately rips open that you offer to her with a large

needle . . . and puts into the vein as much venom as can lie upon the head of her needle. . . . There is no example of anyone who has died of it; and you may believe I am very well satisfied by the safety of the experiment, since I intend to try it on my dear little son. I am patriot enough to bring this useful invention into fashion in England."[13]

Montagu was over-optimistic about the success rate and the risks of the procedure, but she was good to her word regarding both her son and her efforts to popularize the treatment back home. Caroline, Princess of Wales, was daughter-in-law to King George I, who'd come to the throne on smallpox's extinction of the Stuart royal line. In 1720, she was persuaded by her friend Lady Mary to explore inoculating her children. After watching successful experiments on six criminals followed by six orphaned children, she did so. That helped spur growing acceptance of the measure.

Smallpox inoculation may be one reason why survival rates for the children of the British royal family dramatically improved between the seventeenth and eighteenth centuries. About four out of every ten royals born between 1600 and 1699 died before their first birthday. That dropped to one child out of thirty-five in the years between 1700 and 1799. But death rates for babies born to commoners remained broadly unchanged, with about one in four dying before their first birthday.[14] A combination of medical mistrust, expense, and risk (some people caught full-blooded smallpox from inoculation, and perhaps as many as one in fifty died from it) meant both that the treatment's spread was limited and that smallpox remained a major killer.

The invention of a truly safe, cheap, and more reliable vaccination procedure against smallpox was an early step in a series that helped break the world out of the infectious Malthusian trap. It's ironic that the Black Death had a connection with the discovery of that vaccine, which in the wake of the Great Mortality could be found in the observation that women recruited to fill the ranks of animal tenders appeared to be favored when it came to the risk of smallpox infection.

Dr. Edward Jenner made his living as a country doctor, but his scientific interests were broad and voracious. He spent a decade working on his natural history of the cuckoo, published in the *Philosophical Transactions* of the Royal Society, the same journal that had reported on variolation. Jenner's research had involved extensive observations, numerous dissections, posting cuckoo stomachs to London for further analysis, and swapping eggs between nests. That was just one part of a scientific exploration that led to his workroom being filled with such specimens as rooks, swifts, dogs, pigs, a bottlenose dolphin, and numerous hedgehog heads alongside human hearts (Jenner was one of the first to analyze the causes of angina). He became an expert in sexing eels, and constructed an early hydrogen balloon, which he flew over Berkeley Castle.[15]

But it was Jenner's observations on the prevention of smallpox that were to bring him international renown. He noted that many milkmaids had from their wards caught cowpox, a minor annoyance in humans but one that appeared to confer immunity to smallpox. In 1796, Jenner used cowpox lesions from a milkmaid to draw material that he injected into his gardener's eight-year-old son, James Phipps. He then used the technique of inoculation to expose the boy to smallpox more than twenty times. James never developed the mild case of smallpox that usually accompanied inoculation, suggesting he was already immune.

The doctor wrote up his results as *An Inquiry into the Causes and Effects of the Variolae Vaccinae* (Latin for "pustule of cows," from whence the word "vaccine"), published in 1798. While Jenner's contemporary Malthus inevitably suggested the vaccine would make little difference to lives in Europe unless it was coupled with less sex, others were more excited. In 1802, the British Parliament awarded Jenner a prize of 10,000 pounds (followed by twenty thousand more in 1807). Denmark made vaccination compulsory by 1810, followed by Russia in 1812 and Sweden in 1816. Smallpox deaths in Sweden fell from twelve thousand in the year 1801 to eleven deaths in 1822.[16]

Jenner's invention even sparked the first ever globe-spanning public health campaign. In 1803, King Charles IV of Spain shipped twenty-two orphans across the Atlantic on the *Maria Pita*. Vicente Ferrer (aged seven) and Pascual Aniceto (three) were infected with cowpox as the ship sailed, and as the cowpox reached its peak, pus was withdrawn from their poxes and injected into two more children in turn.

Children were used because they were less likely to have been exposed to smallpox already. And the serial process ensured there'd be a child ripe with the pox available to provide the vaccine to American populations after the crossing. At each stop, more children were drafted to support the effort. In Lanzarote "five children of the poor class were sent in order for them to return vaccinated," notes the expedition record. The *Maria Pita* provided vaccines to Venezuela and Mexico. Having crossed to Acapulco, the vaccination campaign recruited a new set of children to continue the cowpox chain across the Pacific. From Manila the expedition spread vaccines to Macau and Canton before returning home.[17]

Taking the Venezuela vaccine strain to South America, Spanish army surgeon Josep de Salvany led the expedition across the Andes to Ecuador. Despite suffering from diabetes, malaria, diphtheria, and tuberculosis, as well as losing both a hand and an eye, Salvany continued the vaccination campaign down through Buenos Aires to reach Bolivia in 1810. There he collapsed and died at age thirty-six. A few days before his death, Salvany wrote that

> the lack of roads, the precipices, the large rivers, the deserted places we have encountered have not stopped us for even a moment, much less the waters, snows, hungers and thirsts we have suffered. The rigors of that cruel contagion offered in our first steps served as stimulus to bring a brilliant purpose to noble and humanitarian tasks.

His poetic self-promotion was surely deserved: overall, 1.5 million people were vaccinated by the campaign. It was a moral failing that the children who'd carried the cowpox across the Atlantic were abandoned in Mexico City's hospice. That said, Jenner was still surely right to call the expedition "a glorious enterprise."[18]

News of Jenner's discovery reached Japan in 1803, the same year that the *Maria Pita* left Spain. But there was no cowpox in the country, so that vaccination had to be imported as it had been to the Americas. The problem: foreign children were not permitted to enter Japan.

Every year between 1821 and 1826, and then again in the 1830s and 1840s, Dutch ships carried bottled cowpox lymph and lancets on the long journey from the East Indies to the port of Nagasaki in Japan, but the vaccination was ineffective by the time it reached its destination. Japanese doctors who'd used variolation understood that smallpox scabs could be preserved, so they asked for the Dutch to send cowpox scabs in 1849. One child was inoculated with the cowpox scabs and developed pocks. Nagasaki city officials brought in children from neighboring communities to be vaccinated and then, arm to arm, they passed on the vaccine to others. By the end of the year, vaccination clinics had been opened across the country.[19]

Jenner's discovery and its adoption saved many millions of lives. In the late eighteenth century in London smallpox accounted for 9 percent of all deaths. By the second half of the nineteenth century that had fallen to around 1 percent.[20] But it wasn't enough to reverse declining health during the early part of the Industrial Revolution. Jenner's work remained a one-off. His breakthrough wasn't based on a fully developed theory of infection or broader experimentation that would allow the benefits to spill over to the creation of other effective preventatives and cures for different diseases.

As a sign of limited progress in broader medical approaches, leech farming became a growth industry in Europe in the early nineteenth century, with leeching the stylish way to partake of bloodletting. Demand reached into the tens of millions of leeches a year.[21] Or look at the treatments given to George Washington as he lay in bed on December 14, 1799, fevered with a throat infection. His medical team drained him of two quarts of blood. They also encouraged him to inhale vinegar and water, gargle more vinegar mixed with sage tea, take doses of mercurous chloride—a laxative—and tartar emetic to encourage vomiting. He was burned to raise blisters and underwent an enema. Washington died on the same day that the doctors had been called.[22]

Regarding the underlying causes of infection, while the germ theory had its adherents, the many different routes taken by microbes to reach a new host helped obscure their role, seemingly contradicting any universal causal theory. Smallpox seemed to demonstrate human-to-human contagion at work, but other diseases did not: yellow fever appeared to spread seasonally, not from person to person (had doctors known it was mosquito-borne, that would have made sense). Both plague (delivered by fleas and rats) and cholera (spread through tainted water) affected the poor more than the rich, suggesting the importance of environment over human contact.[23] This will be one reason why the eighteenth and early nineteenth century saw a distinct recovery of "miasmist" over "contagionist" thinking, especially among the sanitarians who constructed sewer systems to remove smells.

The strength of miasmist belief in the nineteenth century is underscored by the reaction to one medical professional who was partial to the germ theory of disease spread—John Snow. In London's 1854 cholera epidemic, the anesthetist noticed the number of cholera victims who'd used a particular water pump in Broad Street, Soho. He managed to persuade local authorities to remove the pump handle, preventing people from collecting the lethal liquid that poured from it. In evidence to Parliament, Snow explained why the water was so toxic: water closets, filled with cholera germs from victims, flushed human waste into an aging sewer system that leaked into the water supply. Members of Parliament scoffed at the idea: "After careful enquiry we find no reason to adopt this belief." Cholera, they concluded, "multiplies rather in air than in water."[24] (Doubtless many MPs also backed a common treatment for the condition: calomel, a powerful purgative. The supposed cure, which only sped the onset of catastrophic dehydration, was a form of unintentional manslaughter.) Snow died in 1858, his theory still on the fringes of respectability.

German physician Robert Koch's research on anthrax, tuberculosis, and cholera helped turn the tide in favor of the germ theory, as we've seen. His contemporary Louis Pasteur used that knowledge to create the tools for a broad and effective medical response to the threat of infection.

Pasteur himself discovered a number of microorganisms and demonstrated that freshly boiled broth only spoiled if exposed to air, suggesting it was something airborne rather than innate to broth that caused putrefaction. He also showed the role of microorganisms in turning milk sour and wine into vinegar, and the ability to kill those organisms through heating (pasteurization). But Pasteur's greatest contribution to human well-being was to understand the concept that lies behind most common vaccines. That allowed him to take Jenner's one-off miracle and lay the basis for a wide range of cheap immunizations.

Pasteur discovered by accident that old lab-grown chicken cholera didn't kill chickens where fresh cholera samples did. So he tried injecting chickens with old cholera before injecting them with a fresh batch. The chickens stayed healthy. This reminded Pasteur of smallpox vaccination, suggesting that perhaps intentionally "attenuated" (weakened) bacteria could be used to vaccinate people and animals against the disease-causing variant. And he discovered a range of methods to attenuate the chicken cholera: heating, aging, and passing the bacteria through a succession of different animals.

In March 1881, Pasteur demonstrated the same technique with an anthrax vaccine.[25] Four years after Robert Koch first grew anthrax in the lab, Pasteur took anthrax samples and weakened the bacteria through aging and oxidation.

The doctor was nothing if not a showman. Twenty-four sheep, six cows, and a goat were vaccinated against anthrax using the attenuated bacteria he'd developed. A while later, they were intentionally infected with full-strength anthrax alongside a group of unvaccinated animals. Two days after that, Pasteur presented both sets of animals to members of the Agricultural Society of Melun and members of the press.

His vaccinated wards were all still alive. Of the unvaccinated animals, some were already dead, two dropped dead as the crowd watched, and the rest were obviously very sick. Koch wasn't impressed, writing that his French colleague's work was based on luck, and there was nothing new in what Pasteur had done. Those who celebrated him as "a second Jenner" forgot that "Jenner's beneficial discovery was not in sheep but in humans."[26]

But Pasteur's experiment was the start of a revolution: he followed up with a rabies vaccine in 1885, made using the spinal cords of infected rabbits that had been dried for ten days. This he administered to the young Joseph Meister, who'd been repeatedly bitten by a rabid dog and was brought to the lab by his distraught mother. He carried out the experiment with considerably more doubt and trepidation than Jenner reported with regard to his young subject, James Phipps, but Meister recovered—saved an agonizing death by Pasteur's discovery.

Whether driven by jealousy, nationalism, or the perception of legitimate flaws in Pasteur's work, Koch wouldn't relent: he said the Frenchman's results "lack microscopic examinations" and "use unsuitable experimental animals." But thousands of people were saved from rabies within years of the vaccine's creation.[27]

In the 1920s, French researchers used toxins derived from diphtheria and tetanus to create vaccines against those conditions. In 1940, an American researcher used flu virus grown in eggs and then killed with formaldehyde to create a flu vaccine. In the 1950s, Jonas Salk changed the world with his polio vaccine, cultured in monkey kidneys. In the years that followed, Maurice Hilleman, a research scientist at the pharmaceutical company Merck, took a lead part in research and development efforts that produced vaccines against measles, mumps, rubella, chickenpox, hepatitis A and B, pneumococcus, meningococcus, and *Haemophilus influenzae* type B (HiB).[28]

Paul Offit, a noted vaccine inventor himself, described

the approach taken by Dr. Michiaki Takahashi to attenuate the chickenpox virus that Hilleman would turn into a workable vaccine. Takahashi passed a viral sample taken from a three-year-old through fetal cells of both humans and guinea pigs at cold temperatures. The virus that emerged from the process, many generations evolved from the original, was weaker than wild chickenpox, and could be defeated by the human immune system. But it was close enough to the original virus that fighting it generated subsequent immunity to full-bore chickenpox. Prior to the vaccine, 4 million children in the US alone contracted chickenpox each year, and a few unlucky ones among them developed hepatitis, brain swelling, and fatal pneumonia as a result. Since the vaccine, chickenpox mortality in the US has fallen 90 percent.[29]

A second health technology of immense consequence to the fight against infection was the antibiotic—a drug that could kill harmful bacteria. Penicillin was first discovered by Sir Alexander Fleming in the UK in 1929—he found that the penecillium mold produced a substance that killed the bacteria staphylococcus (a cause of pneumonia, skin infections, and food and blood poisoning among other maladies). Subsequently Fleming showed that penecillium was harmless to humans. But the antibiotic wasn't manufactured at scale until the waning years of the Second World War. In 1941, total production worldwide was enough to treat only two hundred patients. By 1949, the US was producing 76,000 pounds of penicillin, and fifteen years later that number had climbed to 1.7 million pounds. The price per pound dropped from $1,114 to $49 over those same fifteen years.[30]

The rollout of antibiotics had a massive impact on infection—from wounds but also contagious conditions. Antibiotics can help treat or cure leprosy, the plague, cholera, typhus, syphilis, and gangrene. In the US, cases of syphilis, already falling thanks to wider acceptance of condoms after Allied militaries finally started issuing them during the Second World War, tumbled from 70 for every 100,000 people to 4 out of 100,000 over just the ten years after 1946. Antibiotic treatment not only cured victims but prevented their future partners and *their* partners from getting the disease. The reduced intercourse risk was one spur for the sexual revolution of the 1960s.[31] And typhus, the disease that had sunk Napoleon's Russia campaign, has been, with the widespread help of antibiotics, limited to mountainous pockets in Peru, North Africa, Ethiopia, and Russia itself.[32]

It wasn't just new medicines; it was the tool of delivery. Some forms of penicillin and most vaccines needed syringes to inject them. And over the course of the first sixty years of the twentieth century, injection technology was also revolutionized. Handmade glass-and-metal syringes cost about $50 each in 1900. Machine technology was developed before the First World War that eventually brought the price down to around $10 a syringe by 1950. The development of mass-produced single-use plastic syringes in the 1950s reduced the price to 18 cents by 1960 and about 1.5 cents by 2000.[33] The smallpox vaccine was eventually delivered with a simple bifurcated needle—two spikes of metal.

When syringes are expensive, they have to be re-used a lot. Between 1917 and 1919, a vaccination campaign in French Equatorial Africa used just six syringes to deliver 90,000 vaccinations against sleeping sickness.[34] That significantly increased the risk that vaccination campaigns would be a source of infection themselves. Not that the problem has completely disappeared in the age of the disposable syringe: a 2014 study sponsored by the World Health Organization estimated that up to 1.7 million people were infected each year with hepatitis B virus, and 33,800 with HIV, through an unsafe injection.[35] Nonetheless, global health has been transformed by cheap delivery mechanisms combined with cheap vaccines.

• • •

The single most important victory against disease was the global eradication of smallpox. In 1801, Jenner had suggested that "the annihilation of . . . the most dreadful scourge of the human species" would be the final result of his invention,[36] but it still took both time and luck. In 1966, the Nineteenth World Health Assembly called for intensified efforts to eradicate smallpox. In a rare case of Cold War cooperation, the USSR donated more than 140 million doses of the vaccine annually while the US provided more vaccines together with advisers and equipment to rapidly roll out elimination efforts across twenty West African countries. In three and a half years, the disease was gone from the region. And the new bifurcated needle made vaccination something that could be carried out by anyone after a couple of hours of training: dip the needle in the vaccine bottle and the right amount would be caught between the twin points.[37]

Nonetheless, Donald Henderson, a participant in the global effort, reports smallpox eradication "was achieved by the narrowest of margins." Progress "wavered between success and disaster, often only to be decided by quixotic circumstance or extraordinary performances by field staff."[38] Because 100 percent global immunization was an implausible goal (even fifty years later, millions of children go without vaccines each year), the campaign relied on reaching sites of infection fast enough that (nearly) all those in the vicinity could be given a shot to stop the outbreak from spreading. Again and again, vaccine teams raced to remote sites and immunized enough people fast enough that smallpox was contained.

In India, even after the World Health Organization thought that all cases of smallpox had been eradicated, the monitoring still went on—and that monitoring operation shows the scale of the global effort to eradicate the disease. In one month, 668,332 villages were searched by 115,347 workers visiting more than 3 million households. The effort uncovered 41,485 cases of chickenpox, but not one of smallpox—and so India was declared smallpox-free.[39]

In 1977, Ali Maow Maalin, a hospital cook from Mogadishu in Somalia, was asked for directions to the hospital by a man with two sick children. Maalin jumped in the van and started giving directions. The father warned him: the children had smallpox. Maalin replied, "Don't worry about that." But he'd long been afraid of needles and had dodged vaccinators. "It looked like the shot hurt," he said. As a result, Maalin caught the disease.

But unlike hundreds of millions of smallpox sufferers in the twentieth century alone—more than five times the number who died in World War Two—he survived. Even better, he was the last person to catch the disease outside of the lab (Janet Parker from the Birmingham lab release was the last to die; her mother had a mild case and recovered). Three years after Maalin was infected, the whole planet was declared smallpox-free. The scourge of the Old World for centuries, and a destroyer of the New World after Columbus, had been completely defeated.

Maalin went on to spend his life vaccinating others. When he met parents who refused to vaccinate their kids, he'd tell his story, Maalin said in 2006: "I tell them how important these vaccines are. I tell them not to do something foolish like me."[40]

In many ways smallpox was a comparatively simple disease to wipe out worldwide. There's no animal reservoir of the infection (bats or birds, for example)—wipe it out in humans and it's gone. Once you've had smallpox or the vaccine against it, you're immune. When you have the disease, it's quickly obvious. That makes a strategy of watching for people to display symptoms and then rapidly vaccinating everyone around them (known as "ring vaccination") an effective approach to stop outbreaks. The same vaccine worked worldwide and it was cheap and stable—it didn't require refrigeration or complex injection. Other diseases *don't* share these features: there's still no malaria vaccine; many people with polio show few symptoms; Ebola has an animal reservoir. Covid-19 is slower to develop symptoms; many carriers have none. And there's an animal reservoir in bats. That's why the complete victory against smallpox has been hard to replicate in the past and would be hard to achieve with Covid-19.

But progress against other infections has been impressive nonetheless. Ali Maow Maalin became a foot soldier in the global fight against polio. "I'm the last smallpox case in the world," he said. "I want to help ensure my country will not be last in stopping polio." And Somalia was polio-free at least for the first three months of 2020.

In 1952, more than 50,000 children were paralyzed by a polio outbreak in the United States alone. In 1981, there were only 65,000 new cases reported worldwide. That number dropped to 628 in 2011.[41] In 2016, one of the three strains of inactivated polio was removed from the vaccine because it had been confirmed eradicated. At the start of 2020, wild poliovirus was limited to the two countries of Pakistan and Afghanistan.[42]

This is only one more example of considerable progress thanks to global vaccination efforts. Currently in use in the US are vaccines against twenty-six different diseases—including anthrax, cholera, flu, measles, polio, smallpox, and tuberculosis. Not all are 100 percent effective, but all offer significant protection.[43] Fifteen diseases are covered by the vaccinations regularly given to children in the US, and increasingly those same vaccines are being given to children worldwide.

At the start of the 1970s, global vaccination rates against tuberculosis, diphtheria, polio, tetanus, and measles were all below 5 percent. By the end of the decade they'd reached nearly 20 percent. Ten years later they were at 70 percent. And by the end of the century, four out of five children worldwide were fully vaccinated. The number has continued to climb.

Vaccinations and antibiotics are part of a broader story. As James Riley's *Rising Life Expectancy: A Global History* lays out, public health, medicine, rising incomes, improved diets, behavior change, and improved education all played a role in improved global health, with relative contributions varying across time and geography.[44]

Take one of the simplest treatments for a major killer, oral rehydration therapy. It was developed by the Indian doctor Dilip Mahalanabis. As a pediatrician specializing in infections of the digestive tract, Mahalanabis was part of a team of researchers studying cures for diarrhea, a mass murderer in India and across the developing world. The condition is the deadly tool of choice for a range of infectious diseases to spread, as we've seen.

Mahalanabis's clinical research was cut short by war. In 1971, East Pakistan—soon to be named Bangladesh—declared its independence from West Pakistan. During the bloody struggle, 9 million refugees fled across the border of East Pakistan into India. Bangaon, in India's state of West Bengal, was home to a refugee camp of more than 350,000 people. Dr. Mahalanabis was put in charge of health at the camp. As was usual in refugee camps at the time, diarrhea was rampant, linked to appalling sanitation. Mortality rates among infected patients were running at 20 to 30 percent.

"When I arrived, I was really taken aback," Mahalanabis recalled. "There were two rooms in the hospital in Bangaon that were filled with severely ill cholera patients lying on the floor. In order to treat these people . . . you literally had to kneel down in their feces and their vomit. Within forty-eight hours of arriving there, I realized we were losing the battle." He had only two staff members capable of administering intravenous drips—bags of sugar-salt solution piped through a needle into the vein of a patient, the standard medical response to acute diarrhea. And supplies for the intravenous treatment were running out.[45] So the doctor tried the approach he'd been researching back in Calcutta.

Mahalanabis found a large drum, filled it with water, added bags of sugar and salt, and stirred. He told family members of diarrhea patients to fill up cans and bottles with the solution and feed it to their suffering relatives until they hated the taste of it.

This "oral rehydration" approach—drinking saline solution rather than "intravenous rehydration" through a needle—could be carried out by anyone with a bucket. It didn't take skilled care or sterile needles. Even clean water was more of a bonus than a necessity. And patients could tell when they'd swallowed enough of the solution to overcome dehydration. Water with sugar and salt tastes like nectar to the dehydrated and like sweetened seawater to the rest of us. Rather than treating the lucky few who reached the clinic before saline drips ran out, using his simple approach Mahalanabis could help sick people all across the camp. Death rates fell from above 20 percent to 3 percent of diarrhea victims.[46]

Since 1971, oral rehydration has become a standard treatment for diarrheal disease worldwide. It's an incredibly cheap and simple response to a massive global killer. But for its full potential to be realized, everyone has to know about it. In the Indian state of Kerala, around 95 percent of parents know it is important to give fluids to a child with diarrhea. In West Bengal—where Dr. Mahalanabis did his lifesaving work over four decades ago—more than half of all parents still give children *less* to drink when they've got diarrhea, which can be a deadly mistake. That's one reason why child mortality is still higher in West Bengal than in Kerala.

Again, understanding that germs cause disease and washing can remove germs is a powerful piece of knowledge not only for doctors but for all of us, even if clean water and quality sanitation are scarce. Cross-country studies suggest that improving the quality of water supplies can reduce diarrhea risk, but providing education in hygiene practices alongside soap can reduce it twice as much.[47]

Toward our goal of fully appreciating how worldwide disease has been reduced, consider the guinea worm, which used to be endemic across Africa, the Middle East, India, and the "Stans" of the former Soviet Union. It has been on the retreat since the 1930s, helped by the crusading efforts of former US president Jimmy Carter, who negotiated the "guinea worm ceasefire" in Sudan in 1995.[48] The break in fighting allowed volunteers to enter the country to work with communities on avoidance and treatment techniques. In the mid-1980s, there were still 3 million sufferers each year, but in recent years the number of infections worldwide is down to below fifty. The approach didn't even take a vaccine or deworming drugs—just people filtering their drinking water through a cloth or sieve and disinfecting or avoiding infected water sources.[49]

Such behavior change has been a vital part of reducing the burden of diseases—from malaria (sleep under a bed net, drain standing water) to HIV (use condoms). It also helps to explain the significant relationship between a mother's education and her child's health outcomes.[50] Kids born to women who have finished primary school are more likely to live than kids born to women who never went to school or dropped out.

Though drugs and behavior change have been crucial, the more widespread use of older anti-infection tools has delivered a contribution as well. Today, more than two-thirds of the world's population uses sanitation services considered "at least basic" by the World Health Organization.[51] A recent program to chlorinate municipal water in Mexico, for example, increased disinfection coverage from just over half to nine out of ten of Mexico's population in eighteen months. That reduced the number of children in the country dying from diarrheal disease by more than a third—saving six thousand lives a year.[52]

Again, people worldwide are eating better, and that makes them less susceptible to infection. The average number of calories eaten by people in Africa each day has climbed from 2,000 per person in the early 1960s to above 2,600 today (although as many as 2 billion people worldwide still don't get enough vitamins and minerals).[53]

But the *true* power of the medical revolution is demonstrated by the considerably improved health outcomes achieved even by people living in extreme poverty without access to improved water and sanitation. Less than one in five urban households in Kenya are connected to the sewage network today, for example. Despite that, infant mortality in Kenya today is around 3 percent—one-third the level in pre-sanitation London.[54]

What unites vaccination, antibiotics, oral rehydration, bed nets, condoms, and water sieves alike is that their cost is very low and they're simple to use. Indeed, while we saw in the last chapter that doctors were a comparatively minor part of the sanitation revolution, the story is only somewhat different in the twentieth century. It's true that the globalization of victory against infection was due in large part to researchers and medical technologies. But the most powerful of those technologies didn't require an extensive network of practicing doctors and hospitals. Even today the number of doctors and nurses in a country still bears a weak relationship to measures of national health like life expectancy or child mortality.[55] If the nineteenth century's progress against infection was largely a victory of engineering and city management, the twentieth century's was mostly about vaccine workers, community volunteers, pharmacists, researchers, and the drug industry.

Between 1900 and 1970, around 70 percent of the decline in mortality in developing countries was driven by lower rates of infectious disease. The biggest contributors were falling rates of respiratory conditions like pneumonia and tuberculosis, where antimicrobial drugs had a huge role to play, and malaria, where better sanitation, bed nets, and quinine-related drugs were effective responses. Since 1970, the drop-off in vaccine-preventable diseases has played a much bigger part thanks to the rollout of immunizations.[56] Plague and typhus, both mass murderers in their day, have now been reduced to the mortality bush leagues. We've seen that no one dies anymore of smallpox, a disease that killed hundreds of millions in the twentieth century alone.[57] Measles, mumps, rubella, diphtheria, pertussis, tetanus—all infect a small fraction of the numbers of decades ago.

That means, worldwide, we've seen a transition to modern forms of death. It started later in the developing world than in rich countries, but it's now far advanced everywhere.[58] In Mexico in 1951, influenza, pneumonia, bronchitis, and diarrhea between them still accounted for nearly one third of all deaths, and other infectious causes added close to another third.[59] In Mexico today, the three leading causes of death are heart disease, stroke, and diabetes.

Sometime in the last few decades, the world as a whole crossed a transition point: for the first time since the spread of civilization (at least), more people across the planet died of noninfectious diseases than from infection. Progress has been rapid: by 2010, infectious diseases accounted for only 11 million out of 53 million deaths worldwide—or just over a fifth of all deaths. Many more people across the planet die from cardiovascular conditions like heart failure and stroke than from all infectious causes combined.[60]

Because infectious diseases strike the (unexposed) young particularly hard, their decline has had the largest impact on child mortality. By the first decade of the twenty-first century, an estimated 2.5 million child deaths were being prevented each year thanks to basic vaccinations alone. Worldwide, in 1800, more than four in ten children born died before their fifth birthday. Even in the richest countries the rate was still above three in ten. Today, the worldwide average is below one in twenty-five.[61]

Across a range of traditions across the planet, a new child remains without a name until it's at least a week old. In Jewish and Islamic customs, circumcision occurs on the eighth day (Leviticus 12:1–8). Ghanaian custom was to wait to name the child until the fortieth day; Ethiopian children got a third and final name only after surviving measles.[62] But, thanks to improved child health, norms are changing.

In the US, more and more parents are announcing the name of their child before it's even born, and holding elaborate baby showers months before the due date.[63] Bill Gates, the Microsoft founder whose charitable foundation has been so pivotal in backing global efforts against disease, has discussed a trip he took to Ethiopia where he met Sebsebila Nassir—a woman who was, herself, named weeks after her birth and who waited a month to name her first child, but who felt confident enough in the survival of her latest child—Amira—to name her immediately at birth.[64] That makes sense—in 1971, almost one-quarter of all kids born in Ethiopia died before their fifth birthday. By the time Amira was born, the corresponding mortality level had dropped to 6 percent.

Looking at overall life expectancy, in 1900, the average person born on planet Earth could expect to live to the age of thirty-three. By 2000, that expectation had doubled. Today, life expectancy is above seventy years—three score and ten.[65] Citizens of the Central African Republic, the world's poorest country, where about two-thirds of the population lives on less than $1.90 a day, have a life expectancy of fifty-one years—which certainly calls for boosting but, as a sign of progress, would have been enviable to most people living on the planet a century earlier.[66]

While developing countries are achieving levels of infectious disease rates that are far lower than those previously achieved by much richer countries, they're also experiencing higher levels of non-infectious risk factors. Death rates from heart disease and hypertension aren't rising solely because infection is on the decline and people have to die of something. It's also that the spread of cheap calories and inactive lifestyles has gone global, too.

In China, more people have jobs where they stand or sit still, and they can afford cigarettes along with a salt-, fat-, and sugar-filled diet including processed foods. As much as half of the country's noncommunicable disease burden is related to such preventable factors.[67] Forty percent of Chinese people aged forty-five to fifty-four are overweight, along with three-quarters of Mexicans and Russians—similar to levels in the US.[68] Nearly 1.5 billion adults worldwide are either overweight or obese.[69] And two out of five Earthlings have elevated blood pressure.[70]

For all the challenges of postindustrial health, and the reality that setbacks such as Covid-19 will continue to emerge, progress against infection has been world-altering. The firestorm of disease set off by civilization has been tamed. For the first time in recorded history, urbanization and globalization are consistent forces for progress in health and quality of life rather than, at best, a mixed blessing and often far worse. And the truly massive health gains have had positive secondary effects vis-á-vis the role of women in society and the labor force, marriage practices, education rates, equality, declining violence, and a shifting global center of economic power.

CHAPTER EIGHT

It's Good to Get Closer

If you had to choose one moment in history in which to be born, and you didn't know in advance whether you were going to be male or female, which country you were going to be from, what your status was, you'd choose right now.

—Barack Obama

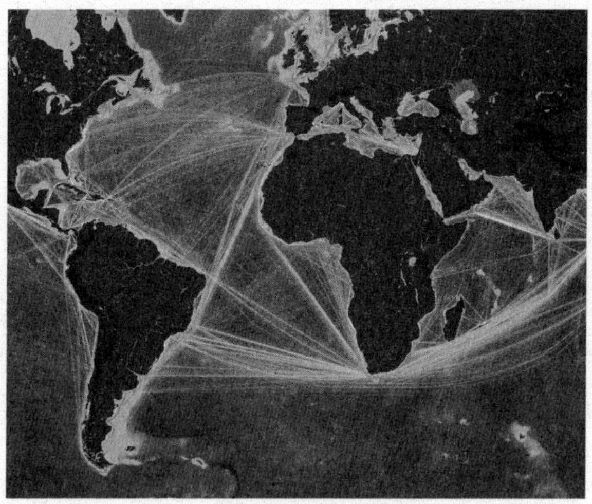

The global merchant fleet (each line is a shipping route) sails free of the delays of quarantine. (Map from shipmap.org © Kiln.digital)

The first stages of the sanitation and medical revolutions ushered in the last great victories of imperialism. While Napoleon's global ambitions were derailed by disease, they were the last to suffer so dramatically: the course of the nineteenth century saw Europeans use infection-fighting tools to preserve their lives long enough to conquer. But globalization at the point of a gun remained bad news for the health of the colonized.

Tropical imperialism relied on all three strategies of exclusion, sanitation, and medication. Exclusion played a role in the theory that whites were primarily—or even exclusively—infected by native populations. The "father of tropical medicine," Sir Patrick Manson, felt that segregation was "the first law of hygiene."[1] Sanitary approaches included draining swamps around towns and camps and moving colonists into hill towns. These were responses to the threat of miasma that (nonetheless) reduced the risk of infection.

Then, in 1820, two French chemists isolated quinine—the active ingredient of fever tree bark that had been traditionally used to treat malaria. Six years later, twenty crewmen of the HMS *North Star* landed in the malarial death zone of Sierra Leone. All but their lieutenant took a daily infusion of fever tree bark in wine, and all but their lieutenant remained healthy. By 1858, the Botanical Gardens at Kew in London was leading a global effort to transport fever bark plants and seeds out of the Andes to plantation sites at Kew, Calcutta, and the Nilgiri hills of India, Singapore, and Java.

And in 1880, enough quinine was being produced to provide 10 million patients with a daily dose.[2] The English rapidly developed a quinine "tonic" water that they drank with gin and lime. It was both more bitter and sweet, as well as considerably warmer, than the version we drink today, providing more evidence of global progress over time.[3]

In 1830, French troops occupied a strip of the North African coastline in modern-day Algeria. Death rates from malaria were initially crippling—as they were among other European troops on the continent—but they began to fall in the face of swamp-drainage and quinine prescriptions. The annual malaria mortality rate dropped from sixty for every thousand people to less than one for every thousand.[4]

Mortality rates for Europeans across the tropics fell even further once the link between mosquitoes and malaria was demonstrated in 1898, and that between mosquitoes and yellow fever was shown by Walter Reed of the US Army in 1900 (the latter thanks to experiments involving brave volunteers who agreed to be bitten by mosquitoes that had recently fed off yellow fever sufferers; the transmission path was demonstrated when they then fell sick themselves). After that, spraying larvicides was added to the mix of interventions against tropical disease.[5]

The result was rapid: in 1875, the year that Henry Morton Stanley started his voyage of exploration down the Congo River, only three European imperial powers had colonies on the continent, largely limited to coastal areas. By 1914, more than 90 percent of the continent had been claimed by colonizers.[6] Algeria alone was home to more than half a million colonists by 1900.[7]

From coastal strips one hundred years earlier, British control extended, by 1914, over the entire Indian subcontinent from modern Pakistan through Bangladesh and Burma down through Malaysia and Papua New Guinea. In Africa, the British Empire occupied a swath of territory from modern Egypt and the Sudans through Kenya, modern South Africa, Zimbabwe, Zambia, and Malawi, as well as Nigeria and Ghana. The American empire expanded as well, critically dependent on mosquito control. Spraying pesticides was an important reason that the US was able to finish construction of the Panama Canal—in contrast to the French, who'd failed a quarter century before after suffering appalling casualties.

In India and Africa, quinine and swamp drainage remained too expensive for European imperial authorities to consider as practical tools for lowering native mortality.[8] Protected colonists behind their *cordons sanitaires*, sipping gin and tonic under the netting, could ignore the death toll and the disease risk of forced labor and mass movement faced by Indians and Africans.[9]

Morton Stanley, explorer of the Congo, was famed for uttering the words "Dr. Livingstone, I presume?" on meeting his fellow explorer near Lake Tanganyika—although he probably made up the quote sometime later for the readers of the *New York Herald*. Stanley was widely reviled for his treatment of African porters—making him a perfect partner for Belgium's King Leopold, whose private empire in the Congo Basin (the current-day Democratic Republic of the Congo) used slavery and violence on a massive scale to tap and export rubber. But the explorer's biggest contribution to misery on the continent may have been an accidental one: spreading sleeping sickness across the heart of Africa.

Sleeping sickness is transmitted by the blood-sucking tsetse fly—which picks up the protozoan parasite along with a meal from an infected human or animal carrier. When it buzzes on to its next unwilling host, the tsetse deposits thousands of parasites into the bloodstream. As they multiply, the victim suffers confusion, mood swings, and overwhelming exhaustion. Eventually the infected person may fall into a troubled sleep, thence to a coma and finally to death.

The sickness had been known in parts of West Africa from the 1300s, and health economist Marcella Alsan argues that its deadly effect on animals was a significant deterrent to agriculture, the development of centralized states, and, through those effects, modern economic performance.[10] But much of the continent (including precolonial empires like Great Zimbabwe) remained infection free until the end of the nineteenth century. The tsetse fly was already there. All that was required was a sufficient number of infected visitors to start up the cycle of sickness.

And in the employ of King Leopold, Stanley provided the hosts. He set up stations along the River Congo in the early 1880s. Explorers, plantation managers, and traders—with their porters and guards—started traveling up and down the river in increasing numbers. By 1904, the *New York Times* reported thirty thousand sleeping sickness deaths in villages around Lake Victoria. The newspaper, focusing on what mattered, declared the disease "a terrible evil that is beginning to oppose a powerful barrier to . . . colonial enterprises in tropical Africa."[11]

In French West Africa, meanwhile, universal conscription and "corvee labor" (temporary enslavement by the colonial government in lieu of tax) ensured the further mixing of disease pools. Voluntary and involuntary migrants died in the tens of thousands as they were exposed to local varieties of infections, including malaria. And returning workers carried the new strains back home, where they killed yet more people.[12]

In India, railroads—and the workers who migrated to build them—spread cholera. Farmworkers migrating to tea plantations spread hookworm, while large-scale rice plantations fostered malarial mosquitoes. Migrant workers in mines were particularly at risk of tuberculosis—and also spread it back to their homes when they returned.[13]

Only with the spread of, first, new technologies of infectious disease control and, second, postcolonial governments at last prioritizing the health of the majority did life expectancies begin to rise in earnest in the developing world. An important dividend was that city living and global travel became safer for everyone. Victories against infection allowed the world to get closer, which proved a vital spur to innovation. But it also radically reshaped demographics, refuting Malthus's predictions about what happens when people get rich and live longer.

With the medical advances of the twentieth century, cities worldwide finally became healthy enough to expand. In many of the world's poorest cities today, most urban population growth is due not to migration but to city residents having children that survive more often. Looking at recent survey data, Nobel Prize–winning economists Abhijit Banerjee and Esther Duflo found that, among the world's poorest—those who live on less than a dollar a day—infant mortality rates in urban areas were lower than rural rates in two-thirds of the countries for which they had data.[14] That slum living in many developing countries is healthier than the rural alternative is a complete reverse of the global situation a century ago.

That helps to account for the global growth of cities. In 1960,

1 billion people lived in urban areas worldwide. Today that's closer to 4 billion—the majority of the world's population. In 1800, Tertius Chandler's city population data reported one city (Beijing) with a population of more than 1 million people. By 1900, that had reached 16 such cities. In 1950, the United Nations listed 77, well under one-half of which were in what might generously be considered the developing world at the time. The UN suggests there were 501 cities with more than 1 million people by 2015, the overwhelming majority in the developing world.[15]

Urbanization has always been a key to economic dynamism. Concentrating economic activity in cities makes it easier to transport goods from producers to consumers. Having many people in the same place allows workers to specialize. Economist Edward Glaeser points to the Yellow Pages: if you want a store that specializes in necktie restoration, you'd better hope you are in a major metropolis. Or if you want a doctor that specializes in rare diseases, look to a place likely to hold enough patients.

And urban areas are the centers of technology advance because entrepreneurs and inventors learn from one another. In the US, 96 percent of new product innovations occur in metropolitan areas, with nearly one-half of the total in New York, Los Angeles, Boston, and San Francisco alone. The advantages of agglomeration also help to explain why workers who live near a city that employs more than half a million people earn a third more than those outside a metropolitan area.[16]

It isn't just the US: the half of the world's population that lives in urban areas generates more than 80 percent of global output, while 600 cities that account for just one-fifth of the global population generate more than 60 percent of global output.[17] Urban living is also healthier for the environment as it tends to involve less travel and smaller housing.[18] Add to that the fact that urban dwellers are ideologically different from their rural counterparts: comparatively liberal, international, trade- and migration-loving, in favor of gender equality and gay rights, environment-defending, and open-minded in matters of religion.[19] The city is progressive—and it's where progress happens.

Just as getting closer allows for greater specialization and innovation within cities, global connectivity allows for specialization and innovation across countries.

To see how much the sanitary and medical revolutions have changed the risks of global interaction, examine what kills Americans abroad these days: cardiovascular events including heart attacks account for 49 percent of all deaths, injuries for a further 25 percent, and infectious diseases other than pneumonia for just 1 percent. Of course, most US travel is to places where infectious disease risk for Americans has long been comparatively low, but even travel to pathogen-rich environments has become far, far safer than it used to be: a study of 185 deaths of US Peace Corps volunteers, placed in some of the world's *least* healthy countries, found that unintentional injuries and suicides were far more deadly than infection, accounting for more than 80 percent of deaths between them.[20]

The same applies to Chinese engineers traveling to Malawi to help build a road or Brazilian executives flying to Laos to ink a commercial agreement. And while outbreaks from cholera to Covid-19 demonstrate travel still spreads diseases, each individual traveler usually faces a very small risk of being the victim—or cause—of a new outbreak. Modern medicine, along with improved sanitation when it is available, has made international travel pretty much as safe as staying at home—a massive change from two hundred years ago.

That has been a huge force behind globalization. We've seen

that high-infection environments foster closed social networks and distrust of strangers. Similarly, declining risk of infection leads to greater openness: for example, psychologist Julie Huang has found that vaccinated test subjects, when they're reminded of disease threats, are less likely to show prejudice against immigrants than unvaccinated subjects.[21] Not surprisingly, when people have few worries about getting sick, they're more willing to travel and trade, welcome strangers, and try new things.

Looking at the US, the total number of travelers taking an ocean journey overseas from America in the year 1820 was around twenty-one hundred—or 0.02 percent of the population. By 1960 (adding in long-haul air flights), that had reached a little less than 1 percent of the population. At the turn of this millennium, the annual number of US international travelers as a percentage of the population was 9 percent, involving nearly 25 million trips a year.[22] Worldwide, in recent years, 1.2 billion people have traveled internationally as tourists each year (2020 will be a tragic exception, of course).[23]

Transport technologies have made travel considerably cheaper, but that level of movement only occurred because the fear of the foreign and the reaction of exclusion was on the decline. Tourists with two weeks' holiday a year would likely be deterred by a quarantine period three times that long, and so would business travelers or scientists headed to an international conference. That's to say nothing of people deterred by the risk that travel would kill them. Plus, permanent migration is easier in a world where infection isn't a reason to exclude. That's particularly good news for health services in rich countries: nearly one out of every three physicians and surgeons in the US is foreign-born, along with a quarter of the health aides, a fifth of the lab technicians, and half the medical scientists.[24]

Safer travel makes it easier for people to scout opportunities, make deals, and set up operations—even in the Age of Zoom. Think of what's involved, for example, in running more than twenty-four thousand Starbucks stores in seventy countries, or managing some other part of the $6 trillion worth of US foreign direct investment worldwide.[25]

The story is the same with trade: it can't happen without global movement of people—sailors, pilots, marketers, and salespeople. In 1820, the United Kingdom exported goods worth $53 per inhabitant. By 2003, that total had reached $5,342—a hundred-fold increase. The corresponding figures for the United States are $25 and $2,762—an even faster growth rate.[26] Nearly 10 million US workers directly depend on exports for their jobs. About one-sixth of everything Americans buy comes from abroad.[27] And the US is one of the least globally integrated countries in the world.

Trade allows countries to *specialize*, including when it comes to medical supplies. For example, the US is the world's largest importer of personal protective equipment: the country imports far more respirators, gloves, and goggles than it exports. But it also exports more hand sanitizers and face shields than it imports.[28] And finished products—respirators or ventilators, for example—are made up of components from lots of different countries. Trade enables the US and the rest of the world to get vital medical equipment at a far lower cost than if everyone produced it all at home. It's why early efforts to restrict trade in that equipment in 2020 were a tragic mistake for everyone.

But trade also allows countries to import things they simply can't produce at home. The United States can no longer be self-sufficient, if it ever truly was. It imports the majority of the cobalt it consumes, for example.[29] And even large economies can't produce enough food in some years and need to import it: trade is a vital part of the story of the global decline of famine over the past century.

Smaller countries often lack the market size or productive capacity to make home production of a whole range of goods feasible. Look at pharmaceuticals: in 2004, the World Health Organization estimated that twenty-seven of the world's countries had the ability to innovate in the production of new drugs, and ten of those had a sophisticated pharmaceutical industry undertaking significant research. Thirteen more countries were manufacturing both active ingredients and finished products. That left 126 countries that either had no pharmaceutical industry at all or relied on imported ingredients for all of their production.[30] Without international trade in pharmaceutical products, those countries would have *no* vaccines and *no* antibiotics. They'd suffer nineteenth-century levels of health. For all that globalization was, in the past, a force for spreading disease, today it's simply central to planetary well-being.

Global connections facilitated by low infection risk have sped innovation, too. Look at worldwide collaboration on the vaccine developed against Ebola in 2015: US players in the research included Yale University, the Army Medical Institute, the Walter Reed Army Institute of Research, and the National Institutes of Health. But also playing a vital role were the Institute of Virology in Marburg, Germany, as well as the German vaccine manufacturer IDT Biologika, the Canadian National Microbiology Lab, and the World Health Organization. And nine separate countries were involved in the clinical trials set up to determine if the vaccine worked.[31]

Nobel Prize–winning economists Michael Kremer and Paul Romer both suggest that, over the long term, there's a simple relationship between the size of a connected population and the speed of technological advance.[32] Small, isolated communities see technological stagnation while large, integrated populations foster rapid innovation. Technological advance is the big reason global quality of life has risen so much over the past two hundred years, and the decline in infection is a big reason for the population growth and connectivity behind that advance. At a global scale, Malthus's fear that more people would lead to greater poverty has turned out to be precisely wrong.

At the same time, while Malthus worried that improved health would only lead to more people living in misery, declines in infection rates have had the—mostly positive—effect of lowering birth rates.

Luis Angeles of the University of Glasgow looked at the data on mortality and fertility around the world over the last few decades and suggests the following pattern: as child mortality declines, the number of children women give birth to declines, too—with about a decade lag. Because of the lag, and because fewer children are dying, the short-term impact of the mortality decline is a growing population. That's why each human only shared the planet with 2.5 billion others as recently as 1950 but now has more than 7 billion potential friends and partners. Over the longer term the trend reverses: as health improves in elder children and adults as well, fertility rates drop further, and population growth begins to slow, or even reverse.[33]

Take the Middle East: In 1960, about one-quarter of children in the region died before their fifth birthday and the average woman gave birth seven times. In 1980, child mortality had halved, while fertility rates remained largely unchanged. But by 2000, fertility had begun a rapid descent to three births per woman. One impact of these changes is that the chance that a woman in the Middle East will watch one of her children die before the age of five has fallen from ubiquity to rarity: about 85 percent would have lost a child in 1960, compared to 10 percent today.

According to the United Nations, the number of children born to the average woman fell from 5.8 to 2.3 in both Latin America and Asia between the early 1950s and the first decade of the new millennium. Africa lagged, but nonetheless the birth rate there fell from 6.6 to 4.9 children over that time.[34]

The decline in both fertility and young mortality has helped age populations. In 1980, the global median age was twenty-three. By 2050, it will be thirty-eight. Work by Harvard's David Bloom suggests there can be a "demographic dividend" during these population changes.[35] After birth rates fall, the proportion of the population that is of working age climbs (because there are fewer school-age children) before it eventually falls (because there are more retirees). More workers and fewer dependents in that middle period allows for higher rates of investment and growth.

But the dividend only pays out if all of those young people have something productive to do. In East Asia in the last decades of the twentieth century, they flocked to factories and manufactured the toys, clothes, and electronics stamped *Made in Thailand* or *Made in China* that were exported to Europe and the US. Bloom suggests that productive use of the "youth bulge" may have accounted for as much as a third of East Asia's miracle growth rates, catapulting countries like South Korea to high-income status and leaving China the largest economy in the world.

Other regions including the Middle East haven't done as well in converting the health revolution into an economic revolution. The few large firms there were kept in business through government contracts and favorable treatment by regulators—not by producing globally competitive products. There's no Middle Eastern equivalent of Hyundai or Lenovo, exporting cars or computers around the world. And so there were few good jobs, but a lot of frustrated job seekers. They had nowhere to go but the street. The lesson for Africa—still undergoing the transition to low birth rates—may be that a well-managed demographic dividend leads to East Asian growth rates, while a poorly managed age transition leads to the Arab Spring and (potentially) its grim aftermath.

As well as producing a bulge in the working-age population, changing demographics mean that women can spend more time in the workplace. In the US, an average woman born in 1900 would be pregnant for more than a third of the time between the ages of twenty-three and thirty-three, and nursing for about a third more. Her compound risk of dying from complications of pregnancy or childbirth was about 3 percent, and more than half of all women suffered some sort of pregnancy- or childbirth-related disablement. Thankfully, risks of serious disablement from a pregnancy are a fraction of that level today—and women are getting pregnant less often. Not surprisingly, that's had a dramatic effect on their ability to work outside the home. Only about 3 percent of married women were in the US workforce in 1890. By 1990, the figure had reached 70 percent.[36] The decline of disease has started to reverse the millennia-long "civilized" subjugation of women.

Not just women benefited from somewhat increased liberty as infection rates fell. Infectious disease risk has long been among the most common reasons—or, at least, *excuses*—to regulate the behavior of both sexes. Across the world, countries where pathogens are more prevalent have a greater tendency to regulate or stigmatize promiscuous behavior.[37] But as infection risk declined, so did the perceived need for some of these strictures. The sexual revolution of the 1950s and '60s followed a period in which infectious diseases—including a number of sexually transmitted diseases like syphilis—had been in retreat for two generations thanks to antibiotics, and against the backdrop of a declining birth rate. Result: a new view that sex could be for fun and bonding rather than just procreation—homosexual and masturbatory sex included. Indeed, the number of countries worldwide where homosexuality is illegal has dropped from 150 in 1960 to 72 in 2017.[38]

Improved health alongside declining fertility has also been a factor behind increased investment in education. Economists Daniel Cohen and Laura Leker suggest that, across countries over the past few decades, adding one year to life expectancy at birth leads parents to send their kids to school for an extra three months.[39] One reason for the link: it makes more sense to invest in a child's education if the child is likely to live long enough to use what they learn.

Sadly, the AIDS epidemic has given us the ability to watch the health-to-education link operate in reverse. Economist Sebnem Kalemli-Ozcan looked at demographic trends in a number of African countries and argues that AIDS has encouraged parents to have more children—to ensure some survive. That forces lower investment in each individual child's education.[40] Between 1985 and 2000, high HIV/AIDS prevalence in countries like the Congo led to the average woman having two more children, and the average child receiving more than a third less schooling, than in African countries that had comparatively low HIV prevalence.

Better health prospects in general can also affect our response to new disease threats. University of Chicago economist Emily Oster demonstrated this looking at how HIV affected sexual behavior among African heterosexual men and US homosexual men. While both groups were at comparatively high risk of the disease, only the US homosexual men altered their behavior in response to risk—reducing the number of partners they had sex with by 30 percent between 1984 and 1988 alone.

Oster suggests the reason is that African men had lower life expectancy, AIDS or no—so they had a lower return to protecting themselves from HIV. She found that richer African men with a higher life expectancy absent the AIDS threat were more likely to reduce their number of sexual partners—their payoff to monogamy was higher. If African men had the pre-HIV life expectancy and wealth of American homosexual men, she suggests, their behavior change would have been as dramatic. Poor health prospects encourage risky health behavior, Oster concludes.[41]

If you're probably going to die from an infection tomorrow, your attitude toward risking your life today in a fight might be more relaxed as well. That suggests that improved health and reduced pathogen stress might also be a factor, among many, in lowering rates of violence in a post-Malthusian world. Global battle deaths in the new millennium are at one-tenth their level in the 1950s.[42]

The overall link from health to wealth and broader well-being isn't simple, immediate, and certain. Considerably improved health, even in some of the world's most benighted spots, hasn't made South Koreas or Singapores out of Niger or the Central African Republic.

What bedevils some countries' development prospects remains stubbornly intractable. For example, there's an active debate among developmental economists as to why tropical regions with their high burden of infectious disease are still poorer to this day. On one side are those who think that the current-day impact of disease is reason enough to expect greater poverty. Scourges such as malaria, diarrhea, AIDS, and dengue impact the ability to work, learn, invest, and so on. Jeffrey Sachs at Columbia University and former US treasury secretary Lawrence Summers at Harvard are two economists who have emphasized the contemporaneous impact of infection on economies.[43]

On the other side are economists, such as Daron Acemoglu and

James Robinson, who emphasize the role of history—the impact of disease on the shape of colonial institutions, and through that on the shape of modern political and economic systems.[44]

Both sides have it right. There's evidence for historical *and* contemporaneous impacts of disease on economic success. Tropical disease has delivered a double burden: a grim history of unequal institutions and a grim present of sickness and death. In connection with that, Harvard's Philippe Aghion points out the obvious: countries that start healthy and grow healthier over time experience far more rapid economic growth than countries that start and stay unhealthy.[45]

Nonetheless, globally, victories over infection have dramatically reduced barriers to connection, increased the number of people to connect with, and ensured that the newly connected have the skills and outlook to make the most of the opportunity. All of that helps to explain why a planet that in Malthus's day was home to a billion people living, for the most part, at subsistence level, is, two centuries later, home to more than 7 billion people with average incomes more than twelve times higher.[46]

Although the final data for 2020 will almost certainly show an increase in global poverty as a result of the Covid-19 depression, the decline in the number of extremely poor people living on less than $1.90 a day—from about 60 percent of the world's population in 1970 to less than 10 percent in 2017—is a sign of the ongoing global transition toward a healthier, wealthier, and happier planet. The rollback of infection hasn't only erased the losses that the average human suffered when civilization spread, it has helped vault mankind to an unprecedented standard of living.

That transition has reshaped the global economic order. For

most of the last two thousand years, the world's two most populous countries, India and China, have vied for the top economic spot. The health and economic divergence that began with the Industrial Revolution left China and India behind, overtaken by Western Europe, Japan, and the US. But with the progress of the last couple of decades there has been dramatic convergence. In 1950, China's economy was a little more than two-thirds the size of the United Kingdom's, and less than one-fifth the size of the US economy.[47] At some point toward the end of 2014, China's output overtook that of the United States and the country became the largest economy in the world.

Just as, over the last five hundred years, the distribution of global infection helped determine which countries were colonized and by whom, in the last fifty years the fight against infection has, once again, transformed the contours of world power.

To be sure, resurgent infection can still do immense harm. That's the risk the world will always confront, most recently illustrated by Covid-19. The risk has three parts: urbanization and globalization are still powerful forces for disease development and spread, our old instincts regarding exclusionary response are only just under the surface, and we're misusing our tools to keep infection at bay. In 2020, we saw all three problems play a role with the spread of the coronavirus and our response to it.

CHAPTER NINE

The Revenge of Infection?

We are now in the throes of a third epidemiological transition, in which a resurgence of familiar infections is accompanied by an array of novel diseases, all of which have the potential to spread rapidly due to globalization.

—Kristin Harper and George Armelagos

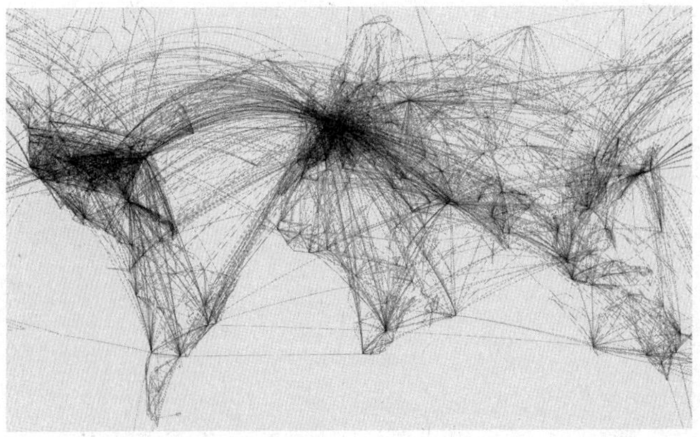

World airline routes. Every (normal) year 1.2 billion people travel to another country as a tourist.
(Credit: Mario Freese)

At the turn of the new millennium, London's population, a shade over 7 million strong, was 27 percent foreign-born, with eighteen different source countries contributing more than thirty thousand residents. Meanwhile, New York's 8 million residents included 33 percent foreign-born, with more than thirty source countries contributing more than fifteen thousand each.[1] Not surprisingly, both are travel hubs: London's Heathrow, Stansted, and Gatwick airports regularly serve a combined 144 million passengers a year, while New York's JFK, LaGuardia, and Newark serve 132 million.

The global metropolises of London and New York have been home to some of the highest average life expectancies and richest people ever. But they were both hit early and tragically hard by Covid-19. They demonstrate both the benefits of a world made safe for connected cities and the costs if we don't keep up our guard against continued disease threats.

In 1855, the missionary Samuel Livingstone came upon Victoria Falls. That discovery marked the end of the great age of land exploration. A century later, humanity regularly traversed every region of the world. It seemed reasonable to assume that the risk of encountering a completely new disease—rather than spreading an old one—would have declined as a result. And in 1962, Nobel Prize–winning virologist Sir Frank Burnet suggested that writing about infectious diseases "is almost to write of something that has passed into history. . . . The most likely forecast about the future of infectious disease is that it will be very dull."[2]

We know it hasn't turned out that way. In fact, even as Burnet was writing, a disease was already circulating in the Congo basin that would shatter predictions of an uneventful infectious future—and within a few years it would spread to the US. On June 5, 1981, the Centers for Disease Control and Prevention in Atlanta issued a new Morbidity and Mortality Weekly Report. The subject was pneumocystis pneumonia, a disease "almost exclusively limited to severely immunosuppressed patients" that had infected five young gay men in the period between October 1980 and May 1981. The cases indicated the possibility of "an association between some aspect of a homosexual lifestyle or disease acquired through sexual contact" and "the possibility of a cellular-immune dysfunction."[3]

These sufferers were getting sick from conditions that implied their immune system—including the white blood cells that are meant to attack invading bacteria and viruses—was deficient. People with healthy immune responses simply didn't get the type of pneumonia these patients had. And whatever had happened to their immune system wasn't a genetic problem, it had been acquired—previously, the victims had been perfectly healthy. By September 1982, when 593 cases of the condition had been reported to the CDC, the disease had an official name: Acquired Immune Deficiency Syndrome.

The human immunodeficiency virus (HIV) was the cause of AIDS. HIV emerged as a mutation from a simian version as long ago as the 1920s, probably in Kinshasa in the Democratic Republic of the Congo. But the first epidemic only occurred fifty years later in Kinshasa, perhaps sadly and ironically helped in its spread by the reuse of needles in immunization campaigns (the virus may have come along for the ride between injections).[4]

When smallpox was eradicated in 1980, AIDS was still unknown as a cause of mortality. But in the early 1980s, outbreaks of "slim disease," the local name for people displaying the symptoms of AIDS, were reported across much of Southern Africa.[5] Only a few years later, in 1989, I spent time teaching in a school in rural Bulawayo in Zimbabwe, and all of the students were encouraged to give blood. The country was one of the first in the world to test all blood donations for HIV, and when the results of that test were passed back to a student in the school, a letter announcing positive status was an invitation to pariah status and death —there wasn't yet any effective treatment.[6]

Just as the Black Death and cholera spread along trade routes, so did AIDS. The University of Chicago's Emily Oster studied the spread of HIV in Africa and found that countries that exported more saw higher rates of infection—with HIV cases concentrated in regions with good road networks. She suggests truckers moving the export goods spread HIV at the same time.[7]

By 1990, AIDS was responsible for around three hundred thousand deaths worldwide a year. And in 2010, the annual death toll was 1.5 million. AIDS still kills as many people yearly as suicide, murder, manslaughter, and war combined. Especially in Sub-Saharan Africa—home to about two-thirds of the world's AIDS sufferers—HIV was a tragic force for reversal in health and broad-based development.[8] Life expectancy in some countries declined by ten years or more thanks to the disease, wiping out decades of previous progress.

Nonetheless, the annual global death toll from AIDS reached a plateau around 2005, and is falling—thanks in no small part to a growing antiretroviral drug industry in developing countries as well as the support of antiretroviral treatments from donor governments including the US.[9] The progress in treatment and prevention has been dramatic, with some hope for an AIDS-free generation in the next decades. In 2013, for the first time ever, fewer people worldwide were newly infected than put on the antiretroviral drugs that keep HIV victims alive and help prevent them from infecting others.

The global response to HIV was unprecedented—too small and two decades too late, but massive and effective in comparison to previous anti-plague efforts. And progress against AIDS is one sign of why we're in a far better place today in the battle against infection than we were fifty, five hundred, or five thousand years ago. The AIDS crisis demonstrated the risk of new threats but also highlighted the potential effectiveness of strong national health systems, research capacity, and coordinated international response to control disease.

The early stages of the Covid-19 pandemic augured a similar combination of slow reaction and opportunities missed alongside the stirrings of a historically unprecedented response. Hopefully, next time, we'll act faster and save more lives. Because the other lesson driven home by the four decades between HIV and Covid-19 is that, thanks to expanding agriculture, dense populations, and global links, there'll be a next time.

Evolutionary biologist Katherine Smith and colleagues at Brown University studied more than twelve thousand reported disease outbreaks worldwide since 1980 and concluded that both the number of diseases and the number of outbreaks have been increasing over time (though the good news is that the cases of illness in each outbreak have declined thanks to better surveillance, prevention, and treatment).[10]

Since 1970, we've seen the emergence of new infections, including severe acute respiratory syndrome, avian influenza, Nipah virus, Hendra virus, Ebola, Marburg fever, Lassa fever, variant Creutzfeldt-Jakob disease, cryptosporidiosis, cyclosporiasis, Whitewater Arroyo virus, hantavirus, and (of course) Covid-19. That's not to mention resurging or reemerging diseases, including multidrug-resistant tuberculosis, monkeypox, dengue and yellow fever, drug-resistant malaria, and even plague.[11]

Some new diseases emerge from forests as HIV did. The 1998 Malaysian Nipah virus epidemic demonstrated how the continued spread of human activity puts us in contact with new zoonotic illness: fruit bats carrying the disease were displaced by deforestation and ended up sharing fruit with pigs crammed into large pens near orchards. As the pigs trampled the fruit bat's droppings, they aerosolized the excrement, and breathed it in. The pigs were infected with the Nipah virus, which was then passed on to human handlers. The condition can cause swelling of the brain, coma, and death—sometimes years after exposure.[12] (Covid-19 likely also emerged from bats.)

Other diseases mutate and evolve from the existing stock of infections that accompany people and their livestock. Humans only reproduce after more—often *considerably* more—than a decade and a half of growth. The average virus produces thousands of offspring in one or two days.[13] That means microbes can evolve a lot faster than their hosts.[14] And even minor mutations can have dramatic implications. Rapid evolution is why previously (comparatively) unthreatening infections can quickly become big killers.[15]

Consider, for example, another recent outbreak: in the week

of April 13, 2009, two unrelated children in Southern California fell ill, coughing, sneezing, and running a temperature. Both sets of parents took them to separate clinics. Both children were tested and found to have flu of an unidentified strain. The children went home with the usual assortment of drugs and both felt better within a week. But according to standard protocols, the United States Centers for Disease Control was alerted. On April 17, four days after the children had visited clinics, the CDC declared that the children had contracted a previously unknown flu virus, swine influenza A H1N1. It was labeled swine influenza because this was a strand that had jumped species from pigs to cause illness in humans. "Concern exists that . . . a large proportion of the population might be susceptible to infection, and that the seasonal influenza vaccine . . . might not provide protection" against the swine influenza variant, reported the CDC.[16]

By the end of the month, the World Health Organization had declared a global pandemic of swine flu. Mexico, at the epicenter of the outbreak, reported 949 laboratory-confirmed cases, including 42 people who'd died of the disease. The country closed schools and banned large public gatherings.[17] By the first week of May, a total of twenty-one countries had reported cases across Asia, Europe, and the Americas. Despite the development of a vaccine to fight the flu strain, deaths from influenza shot up—one estimate is that the pandemic caused 12,469 deaths in the US alone by April 2010.[18]

The risk of infection from livestock has been magnified by factory farming. While "only" 376 million pigs were slaughtered worldwide in 1961, by 2012 that number had climbed to 1.4 billion.[19] And the pigs are grown in increasingly massive lots. The average pork producer in the United States owned fewer than fifty hogs in 1964. Today, that producer owns more than eleven hundred.[20]

Big farms that produce most of the pork and bacon we consume are a multiple of that size. It isn't just pork: the number of chickens worldwide has climbed from 3.9 billion in 1961 to 21.7 billion today. More than three-quarters of all chicken is factory-farmed.[21]

Though the very existence of such farms is, in part, a sign of our success in controlling livestock disease, these operations still expand the space for viruses and bacteria to evolve new threats. Take Malaysia's Nipah outbreak: the country saw dramatic economic growth in the 1980s, and rising incomes increased demand for meat. Malaysia's agricultural sector scaled up massively, replacing family production with factory farming. With thousands of pigs packed into close quarters, a disease that previously jumped from bats to pigs in isolated cases multiplied in sheds of a thousand-plus hogs—and then spread to humans.

The Malaysian government responded by killing 1 million pigs in a mass cull, and Nipah retreated. But it has re-emerged across Asia since then, and it also appears to have become more deadly, killing up to 70 percent of infected pig populations and sometimes spreading directly from one human to another.[22]

And diseases that jump from animals to humans are far more likely to escape the farm or forest village because the world is more connected than ever before.[23] A single crowded New York subway car can hold about 250 people. Through much of history, the great majority of humans have lived in communities no bigger than that. And in an age before motorized transport or decent roads, many people barely left their village. We've seen that this tendency to stick close to home was a protection against the spread of epidemics and pandemics, including the plague.

But not even the poorest people on the planet today travel so little anymore. In 1960, there were around 122 million vehicles on the world's road network. Today, there are about ten times as many vehicles, and the road network is far more extensive, especially in developing countries.[24] With a human population at least 250 times that of four thousand years ago, some living in cities more than five hundred times the size of Ur at that time, diseases are far more likely to find new hosts before they burn out.

Over longer distances, the old mechanisms of disease spread have sped up as well: in August 1519, a flotilla of four Spanish ships under Ferdinand Magellan set off on the first circumnavigation of the globe. In September 1522, three years later, one of the ships made it back into home port. In 1873, Jules Verne published the novel *Around the World in Eighty Days* in which Londoner Phileas Fogg travels via Suez, Bombay, Calcutta, Hong Kong, San Francisco, and New York to arrive back home. And sixteen years later, Nellie Bly, a reporter for the *New York World*, actually managed the feat for real in seventy-two days. In 1976, a Pan Am 747 carried ninety-six passengers around the world in forty-six hours. Give or take, that's one-five-hundredth of the time of the Magellan expedition.[25]

When tourists can travel around the world in a day or two, so can their diseases. If the origin story relating to Columbus's crew is correct, syphilis was record-setting in the 1500s for making it from the Americas to India in only six years. Five hundred years later, microbes were taking round-the-world tours in weeks rather than years. In 2002, severe acute respiratory syndrome, or SARS, emerged in the wet markets of Guangdong Province in China, where live animals are sold to be eaten. It had jumped species from one of those animals—possibly the Himalayan civet cat.[26] Three months later, a doctor from the province who'd contracted the disease spent one day in a Hong Kong hotel during which he infected sixteen guests. Three of them traveled by plane to Toronto, Singapore, and Vietnam. Within weeks the infection had reached eight thousand people in twenty-six countries across five continents.[27]

And in late 2019, Covid-19 may have spread via a Chinese wet market as well. On December 30, the Wuhan city government began to track cases, and on January 5, 2020, a Shanghai lab detected the cause as a novel coronavirus. The first death was recorded on January 11. By the 13th, a case was confirmed in Thailand and by the 20th there was a case in the US. By January 31, there were a total of around ten thousand reported cases in twelve countries.[28]

Given how many infections we share with animals, how many animal diseases may be only a few mutations away from infecting humans, and how rapidly viruses and microbes in particular can mutate and then spread in a connected world, new global pandemics will surely continue to hurl themselves at humanity.

Ronald Barrett and colleagues from the Department of Anthropology at Emory University in Atlanta have gone as far as to suggest that the emergence and re-emergence of disease threats owing to globalization and antibiotic resistance is a sign that we're entering a "third epidemiologic transition" comparable to the rise of infection at the dawn of civilization and its fall in the last century and a half.[29] That (hopefully) goes too far, but it certainly suggests the scale of the risk we need to confront. The fight against disease made our modern, urban, and connected world possible—but it didn't remove the risk that agriculture, urbanization, and globalization have always presented when it comes to new infectious threats.

If the risk of new infection is still a major concern, so is our reaction to that risk should it emerge. Because our earliest instincts regarding infection are increasingly ill-matched to a connected world.

As we saw with smallpox in Japan, new or irregularly occurring diseases in particular can spark fear and the exclusion instinct.

Flu may kill far more people every year than Ebola ever has, but unless we give a new variant a new name (*swine* flu, as it might be), it doesn't raise as much concern. This may help explain why a November 2014 survey in the US ranked Ebola as the third most urgent health problem facing the country—just below the cost of healthcare and ahead of cancer and heart disease. That fear was accompanied by widespread calls for travel bans, even though there'd been only two cases of Ebola transmission inside the United States, neither of which were fatal, and all experts were saying there was little risk of spread.[30]

Again, we've seen that the exclusion instinct is based on evolutionary reality. Staying away from strangers is a rational reaction in the face of an unknown infectious threat. If it isn't clear who is sick, the only strategy that works is to reduce contact with *everyone*.

Today, though, when most of the world lives in cities and only a small minority of the planet's population is in any way self-sufficient when it comes to producing food (or anything else), total isolation simply isn't an option. Testing and isolating the sick, along with tracing their contacts, was a successful strategy against Ebola in 2014 and against Covid in 2020. "Social distancing" was a necessary but expensive fallback in 2020 when we didn't know who was infected.

Distancing and stay-at-home orders worked to reduce the average number of people infected by each person with Covid-19 to below one, meaning that infection rates decreased. But an early estimate of the effects of the coronavirus lockdowns on the US economy from just the one month of April 2020 suggests an average cost of $5,000 per household. (The effects were far larger for some families: more than 20 million people were thrown out of work in the US during April alone.)[31]

And the associated health impacts of the early coronavirus response were considerable worldwide. Those with conditions other than Covid-19 were kept away from hospitals, routine immunization programs were paralyzed, and millions were sunk into poverty where they suffered from malnourishment and the illnesses that are its by-product. Early estimates suggested that in some developing countries the response to Covid-19 might kill more than the infection itself.

Lockdowns were never designed to be a stand-alone solution. Rather, they were a short-term strategy to buy time for better strategies and to prevent hospitals from being overwhelmed by patients. And it's worth repeating that people sensibly and instinctually want to stay away from others when there's a new disease spreading with no cure. At the start of Covid-19's spread, it didn't take regulations from above for people to stop going to restaurants and cut back on shopping. But for whatever highly contagious, often asymptomatic novel infection that comes next, every country needs to be efficient at using the time provided by lockdowns to come up with less restrictive methods to slow spread and build confidence. Those methods should include mass testing and tracing that allows for selective isolation.

Notably, exclusion at the border is far more expensive and far less effective in a world based on global exchange. Quarantines and border controls probably helped reduce the spread of plague, but they proved considerably less useful against cholera and yellow fever in the nineteenth century. Today, even while isolation of the individual sick tourist can be a practical emergency strategy, and short-term travel bans may sometimes have a role to buy extra time to respond to a new pandemic, the world is simply too connected for even the greatest build-a-wall fantasist to think diseases can long be kept out by closing borders.

In 1986, for example, AIDS was added to the list of infections that would prohibit permanent entry under the US Immigration Act. Even tourists with HIV had to apply for a waiver that, if granted, involved an indelible stamp in their passport announcing to all their HIV status. This despite the fact that in 1987 the World Health Organization had concluded that screening or banning international travelers wasn't an effective tool to reduce the HIV burden. You can tell that travel limits didn't work to stop the spread of AIDS because it was first identified in the US (rather than in the Congo Basin) and quickly reached the countries most cut off from international travel and commerce, including Burma under the Junta.

Similarly, travel controls put in place over the H1N1 virus led to a 40 percent drop in air traffic to and from Mexico following the international alert, but had no effect on the spread of the disease. Epidemiologist Paolo Bajardi and colleagues argue that the evidence from the H1N1 outbreak suggests that even a comprehensive travel ban would, at best, have delayed the spread of the condition by twenty days.[32]

The limited efficacy of travel bans in the face of a frequently asymptomatic and rapidly spreading disease was on full display with Covid-19. While it's good to avoid people congregating in airports or in airplanes as much as it is in trains or factories during efforts to reduce the spread of a disease, there's no cross-country evidence that countries that introduced travel bans saw lower rates of coronavirus infection in the first few months of 2020.[33] Early estimates of the overall impact of travel bans suggest they slowed the spread of the virus from between two to three weeks at maximum and zero days at minimum.[34]

The US government issued its first partial travel restrictions on January 31. In the time between the coronavirus emerging in China and the United States travel ban, 390,000 people flew from

China to the US. There's some evidence that Covid-19 may have spread during the Las Vegas Consumer Electronics Show between January 7 and 10, attended by 170,000 people.[35] There was a coronavirus case in the US on the 20th of January. And there was at least one Covid-19 death in California on February 6, suggesting an infection two weeks prior.[36]

Even in the two-month period *after* the US travel ban was introduced, a further 40,000 people (including US citizens and green card holders) made the journey from China to the US.[37] Worldwide, between January and early April, nearly 11 million people flew into the US from countries with confirmed cases of Covid-19.[38] And the threat of wider travel bans meant that millions of people rushed home before they were enforced. That led to packed immigration and customs halls, crushing thousands of people together in a small space for many hours. Crowded terminals at JFK and Newark were likely a factor in the severity of the outbreak that hit New York City.[39]

It wasn't just the US, of course: a French hospital treated someone for pneumonia at the end of December 2019. Blood taken at the time was later tested for Covid-19 and came back positive. France imposed a travel ban in mid-March.

For a globally connected country, there may have been some benefit from imposing travel restrictions in early January or before, but no government acted that early. The first government worldwide to put in place an international travel ban related to Covid-19 was the Marshall Islands. It was introduced on January 24.[40] (That said, small island nations are where short-term travel bans may make the *most* sense: New Zealand banned foreigners entering the country in mid-March 2020 when it had twenty-eight confirmed cases of Covid-19, and put the whole country in lockdown soon thereafter. When that was combined with a vigorous test-trace-isolate strategy for suspected cases, the initial outbreak was rapidly controlled.)[41]

Worse, travel bans remained in place long beyond any hope of efficacy. US bans were in place through the first half of 2020 despite the fact that the country had more confirmed cases of Covid-19 than any other for most of that time.

Banning travel usually simply complicates authorities' response to new disease threats—slowing the arrival of staff, supplies, and equipment to the countries battling an outbreak. Trade and collaboration, the transfer of goods, people, and ideas, are central to supporting health systems as well as developing and rolling out tests, treatments, and cures. We cannot respond effectively alone. We have to respond collectively.

And in the longer term, there are reasons to think travel bans may further increase risk: a 2006 study of HIV-positive travelers from the UK to the US who were taking antiretroviral drugs at the time found that the majority traveled illegally rather than report their condition and risk either exclusion or exposure. Nearly a fifth of those surveyed stopped or delayed taking their antiretroviral medicines for fear of being searched on arrival in the US and their status being discovered.[42] Not only did they increase their own health risks by doing so, given that antiretrovirals help reduce transmission of HIV, the suspension of self-treatment increased the risks to anyone they had sex with in the United States.

Because of the importance of global connections to the quality of life, by far the largest *economic* cost of many recent global infectious threats, including Covid-19, has been the reaction of people and governments to the threat, rather than the disease itself. We've seen that the Black Death could kill off a third of the European continent and the immediate social and economic effect was surprisingly limited. And in an age where travel and trade were a very minor component of the global economy, regulations governing the movement of goods and people were comparatively minor disruptions to local economies. When Dubrovnik was introducing the concept of quarantine to the world, global trade was a few percentage points of output at most.

But the extent of global integration today explains why even fairly insignificant disease threats can have such outsize economic impact. SARS killed fewer than eight hundred people, for example, but the economic cost of the global response was $140 billion.[43] A World Bank estimate from a few years ago of the global costs of a severe global pandemic on the scale of the 1918 flu was that it might equal 5 percent of global gross domestic product, or $3 trillion.[44] Covid-19 quickly showed that estimate to be wildly optimistic.

And because we're no longer in a Malthusian age, pandemics don't even have the small silver lining of fostering equality. Research on epidemics over the last twenty years by economists at the International Monetary Fund suggests that poor people aren't only more likely to die during an outbreak, they're more likely to lose jobs and fall further behind the incomes of the rich.[45]

Long-term exclusion and border controls were always a partially effective response to disease threats, at best. Today, they're simply unaffordable—significantly counterproductive for health, ruinous for quality of life. The only solution is to use the immense innovative power and production capabilities that a globally connected and urbanized world has bequeathed to develop and roll out more effective responses.

An approach based on rapid development and delivery of tests, treatments, and cures would significantly reduce future concern over new diseases, as it has in the past, even with the most deadly of infections. One result of the third plague pandemic (the latest appearance of the Black Death) is that every continent is a home to at least some wild rodents that carry the plague bacillus, including the Western region of the US, for example. There were four cases of human infection in America in 2012.[46] But we haven't put a wall along the eastern edge of the Mississippi to keep out potential carriers of the Black Death. Why? Because we have a vaccine, and (usually) the bacteria can be killed by a course of antibiotics.

But the world still reacts poorly to new disease threats. Rather than deal with the risk before it emerges, through better sanitation and stronger health systems—or, as it happens, through better surveillance, screening, isolation, and research—we respond late and in panic, often with unnecessary acts of cruelty and abuse of human rights. Yet again in 2020 we learned that if we fail to improve on that performance in a globalized and urbanized world built on exchange, we pay an immense price.

CHAPTER TEN

Abusing Our Best Defenses

I have also found that regressive behavioral disorder (RBD) in children is associated with measles, mumps and rubella vaccination.

—Andrew Wakefield

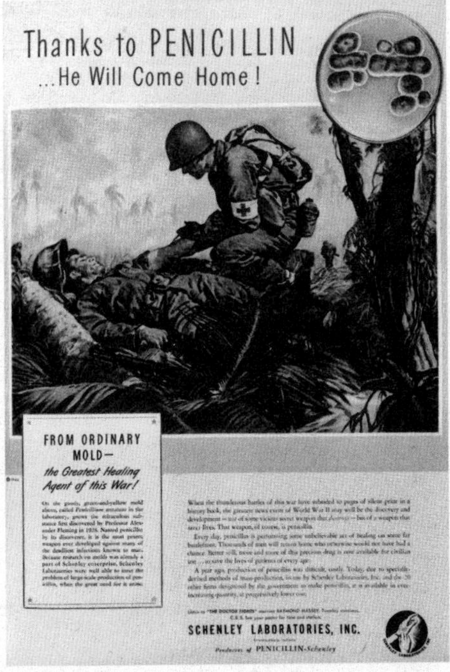

Advertisement for penicillin from *Life* magazine. (Credit: Science Museum, London. Attribution 4.0 International [CC BY 4.0])

In August 2015, pediatricians in Recife on Brazil's Atlantic coast reported a series of disturbing births involving microcephaly—children born with abnormally small heads. Microcephaly can lead to developmental delay, intellectual and learning disabilities, and problems with movement, hearing, and sight. The cause was a virus—Zika—transmitted by the *Aedes aegypti* species of mosquito. The Zika virus is a minor annoyance to those who aren't pregnant; it merely causes joint pain, bloodshot eyes, and headaches. But at least this strain of the virus could cause severe damage to fetuses if it infected a pregnant woman. In response, the World Health Organization told pregnant women not to travel to countries where Zika was circulating. Further, it warned all women to avoid unprotected sex with men who'd visited countries with a Zika outbreak.[1]

Rio de Janeiro was host to the Olympic Games in the summer of 2016, and there were increasingly heated calls to postpone the games or move them somewhere else. But there were good reasons to think the risk to visitors wasn't that large; it was winter in the Southern Hemisphere and Rio was far from the epicenter of cases. The World Health Organization agreed the games should go ahead, and in the end, they did. Not a single case of Zika has been linked back to participants or spectators.[2]

After the games, herd immunity (resistance to the spread of a contagious disease that results when a sufficiently high proportion of individuals in a population are immune to it) dramatically reduced spread: Brazil had 205,578 probable Zika cases in 2016 but only 13,253 by the end of July in 2017, all of which occurred prior to May.[3] Since then, there've been few cases. This was an example where overreaction to a disease threat could have been far more damaging than the threat itself.

But there was a time not too many decades ago when Brazil would have been *completely* free of risk. In 1955, using the insecticide DDT and other control techniques, Brazil eliminated the *Aedes aegypti* mosquito that transmits Zika. The country was re-infested by the end of the 1970s, and soon thereafter dengue fever—also transmitted by *Aedes aegypti*, and frequently the cause of joint pain, bleeding, and in serious cases shock—returned, too.[4] Now there is a growing risk of the return of yellow fever, which uses the very same species of mosquito to spread. Worse, the insecticides commonly deployed against the *Aedes aegypti* have become less and less effective over the past ten years.[5]

Aedes aegypti demonstrates that while we've made immense progress against old infections and their carriers over the past eighty years, it hasn't all been one-way. In an era when we're racing toward eradication of some infections, we're simultaneously abusing our existing weapons against communicable disease so badly that we create new threats. Millions still die prematurely from preventable diseases, in part because we're underutilizing sanitation and vaccination while overusing antibiotics, and we're intentionally developing new diseases as weapons.

• • •

Infectious diseases are still responsible for two-thirds of child deaths worldwide, around one-quarter to one-third of all deaths every year in poorer countries, and around one in twenty of all deaths in the United States in a normal year.[6] Meanwhile, each year, malaria kills almost three times as many people as suffer murder or manslaughter, and diarrheal diseases cause eight times the global death toll from war.[7] And while vaccines and immunizations may avert between 2 and 3 million deaths a year worldwide, 1.5 million children still die each year from vaccine-preventable diseases.[8] This all suggests we have a long way to go in achieving the victories over disease that could be accomplished with existing tools and technologies.

Look at sanitation: 1 billion people worldwide still defecate in public, 2.5 billion lack access to a decent toilet, and 800 million to clean water.[9] Excreting in the nearest field because of inadequate or absent toilets has been a particular problem in densely populated India. In 1925, Mahatma Gandhi complained of his country that "the cause of many of our diseases is the condition of our lavatories and our bad habit of disposing of excreta anywhere and everywhere." Surveys suggest that for every square kilometer in the country there are around 180 people going to the toilet outside—compared to less than half that in the next most feces-burdened countries of Haiti and Nepal. As a result, children regularly catch diseases of the digestive tract that leave them sickly and stunted. Sixty-five million Indian children under the age of five are extremely short for their age. That's a higher proportion of stunting than in far poorer, less stable countries like the Democratic Republic of the Congo or Somalia.[10]

Use a condom, sneeze into your arm, use the toilet, and wash your hands afterward—across the world, even people lucky enough to have access to the necessary infrastructure sometimes don't follow these simple and powerful strategies. In flouting these prescriptions for a less infectious life, they harm themselves and create risk for the rest of us.

And, sadly, the same applies to medical technologies: all too often people don't avail themselves of the most effective treatments or—as bad—misuse those treatments. Not least, conspiracy theories have played a role in keeping the numbers of the unvaccinated higher than they should be, tragically delaying the total extinction of polio, to cite just one example. Making matters worse, some of those conspiracy theories contain an element of truth.

The history of anti-vaccination movements is as old as the technology itself. The 1867 Vaccination Act in the UK, which threatened imprisonment to parents who didn't immunize their children, stirred particularly heated opposition, including the National Anti-Compulsory Vaccination League created in 1874 and the London Society for the Abolition of Compulsory Vaccination in 1879. William White, first editor of the London Society's magazine *Vaccination Inquirer*, suggested that, from Jenner onward, the pro-vaccine camp had dissembled, lied, fabricated evidence, and hidden the truth about the efficacy and safety of vaccination. "Over and over again," he said, "it has been proved that vaccinated patients dead of smallpox have been registered as unvaccinated." Meanwhile, he argued, the elevated death rates of those who'd been given the vaccine had been covered up.[11]

Eight years after smallpox vaccination finally arrived in Japan, an opponent claimed that only one out of ten doctors was in favor of the technique. Practitioners of traditional medicine viewed smallpox as the eruption of an innate poison present since birth rather than an infection.[12] Again, in British India at the height of empire, some saw smallpox vaccination as a plot to poison the Hindu population. Gandhi, right on toilet use, was very wrong on vaccines:

> We are all terribly afraid of the small-pox, and have very crude notions about it. . . . In fact it is caused, just like other diseases, by the blood getting impure owing to some disorder of the bowels. . . . The superstition that it is a contagious disease [has] misled the people into the belief that vaccination is an effective means of preventing it. . . . Vaccination is a barbarous practice, and it is one of the most fatal of all the delusions current in our time.[13]

The imperial authority's response to local opposition was to limit vaccination campaigns to big cities, and even that on a fairly ad-hoc basis.[14]

In the last few years, doctors who should know better have continued an assault against vaccination. In 1996, Dr. Andrew Wakefield, based at the Royal Free Hospital in London, met with a personal injury lawyer, Richard Barr. The lawyer represented parents of a number of autistic children and had been intrigued by Wakefield's writing suggesting that there might be a link between the measles vaccine and Crohn's disease (which causes abdominal pain, anemia, and fatigue). Barr wanted Wakefield to find a link between the measles vaccine and autism, and signed him to an $80,000 contract. Wakefield set to work on five of Barr's clients, who, two years later, would be the majority of eight autistic children featured in an article he published in the *Lancet* medical journal. That article suggested there was a link between the measles-mumps-rubella vaccine and damage to the intestinal wall that allowed harmful proteins to reach the brain, causing autism.

Wakefield didn't compare autism rates among vaccinated and unvaccinated kids, nor name the proteins involved, nor how the vaccine might have caused damage to the intestinal wall. He also didn't mention his contract with Richard Barr, or the fact that Barr had introduced him to his test subjects.

In the years that followed, fourteen separate groups of researchers evaluated the records of more than six hundred thousand children, looking for an autism-vaccination link. Unlike Wakefield's study, the results were convincing, clear, and repeated: no link existed. The Wakefield paper should never have been published and was eventually retracted. But it had an impact nonetheless. In the months after the paper came out, one hundred thousand parents in the UK chose not to vaccinate their children. In Swansea in the UK, one-third of the population went unvaccinated against measles and more than twelve hundred people were infected in an outbreak.[15] Measles returned to France, where an outbreak led to five thousand hospitalizations and ten deaths. Vaccination rates fell in Ireland, too, and three children died as a result.[16]

Dangerous ignorance with spillover effects quickly crossed the Atlantic. Talk show host Jenny McCarthy joined forces with US congressman Dan Burton of the House Committee on Government Reform to expose the supposed autism-vaccination link, and vaccination rates dropped. That has occurred even in some of the world's most technologically literate places—parts of Silicon Valley saw some of the lowest child vaccination rates in the Western world. And in Los Angeles, thousands of parents sent their kids to private schools clutching "personal belief exemption forms," which stated that the child hadn't been immunized for fear of the health impacts that might follow.

Health impacts *have* followed, but they're from the children remaining *unvaccinated*. The schools, some of which had vaccination rates at below 40 percent (the level in South Sudan), have been the epicenter of outbreaks of measles.[17] More than one-half of the 1,416 cases of measles in the US between 2000 and 2015 were among the small minority of people country-wide who were unvaccinated.[18] Ten children died from a whooping cough outbreak in 2010 in California that spread thanks to reduced vaccination rates against that disease.[19]

As in the UK, the anti-vaccination movement in the US was enabled by doctors. LA County pediatrician Jay Gordon advised holding off all immunizations until children are at least three on the grounds that parents had told him "their child has been harmed" by the measles-mumps-rubella vaccine. This while he admitted there was "no evidenced-based medicine, there's no research saying that." In neighboring Orange County, Dr. Bob Sears responded to the measles outbreaks by suggesting there was nothing to worry about: "Ask any Grandma or Grandpa (well, older ones anyway) and they'll say 'Measles? So what? We all had it. It's like chicken pox.'"[20]

In part thanks to Wakefield, Gordon, Sears, and their fellow travelers, vaccine denial has seen a strong resurgence worldwide. Forty-five percent of French survey respondents worry that vaccines are unsafe, alongside 31 percent in Japan. The global proportion is 13 percent—more than one in ten.[21] If more people start acting on their fears and doubts, old infections could come roaring back.

It isn't just the vaccine deniers and their unfortunate children who'd be harmed: some people really can't be given vaccines and they'd suffer the consequences from circulating infections. When she was two, Ashley Echols had a kidney transplant. As part of the transplant procedure, children are given drugs that suppress their immune response so that the body doesn't reject the transplanted organ. As a result, she couldn't complete the standard vaccination regimen. Had Ashley taken the chickenpox vaccine in her weakened state, she might have contracted chickenpox from it. And because of her suppressed immune system, the condition would have been life-threatening. But in June 2017, eleven-year-old Ashley was exposed to a child with chickenpox in Atlanta. So she was rushed to the hospital emergency room to be injected with immunoglobulin. Camille Echols, Ashley's mother, shared the story on Facebook. She ended her post saying "She has been through *so* much already. And this was avoidable."

Thankfully, Ashley didn't contract chickenpox and was fine. But as the number of people who are immuno-suppressed climbs thanks to transplants, treatments against cancer, and diseases including HIV, the risk of the unvaccinated to others will increase. A (dated) estimate suggests there are at least 10 million immunocompromised people in the United States alone.[22]

The parents who choose not to vaccinate their children are not uncaring monsters. They are acting in what they see as the best interests of their loved ones. Vilifying them won't help. But there's a place for legally obliging vaccination, and there should be no tolerance for doctors who risk public health by pandering to conspiracy theorists.

The international effort to eradicate polio has also suffered at the hands of vaccine deniers. In 2003, the governor of Kano state in Nigeria warned that polio vaccines would sterilize recipients—that they were part of a US conspiracy to depopulate the developing world.[23] Polio rates in the country increased fivefold between 2002 and 2006. The Nigerian strain spread to re-infect countries that were previously polio-free. More recently, the opposition to vaccination spread to Pakistan. It began in 2007 with the assassination of the head of polio eradication in the north of the country, who died a victim of the theory that the vaccination campaign was designed to sterilize Muslim girls.

Violence dramatically picked up in 2012, after Taliban leaders called for a jihad against all immunization workers. More than sixty polio vaccinators and security personnel in the country were killed between December 2012 and April 2014.[24] Salma Farooqi was one victim. On the 22nd of March 2014, she spent the day walking through Khyber Pakhtunkhwa province, vaccinating children against the crippling disease. On the night of the 23rd she was back home, asleep with her husband and children in their house in Peshawar. Militants stormed the house, beat her husband, and tied up the children. Salma was dragged from her bed, tortured, and shot, and her body dumped in a field a few miles from her house.[25]

As a result of the violence and intimidation, polio infections doubled between 2009 and 2011 in Pakistan, and a polio virus strain originating from the country was discovered in sewage samples collected as far away as Cairo. From only three countries seeing infections a few years previously, polio cases were reported in ten countries in 2014, including Syria, Iraq, and Egypt.[26]

One factor behind that 2012 surge in violence against vaccinators was the Global War on Terror. In 2011, CIA agents closing in on the location of Osama Bin Laden hatched a scheme to trace the terrorist's DNA. They hired a Pakistani doctor, Shakil Afridi, to orchestrate a hepatitis B vaccination drive in Abbottabad and collect the needles. DNA from the blood in the needles could be compared with a sample from the Al Qaeda leader's sister, who'd died in Boston in 2010. The vaccination team was admitted to the Bin Laden compound, but the operation nonetheless failed—for reasons that remain classified.

The CIA-backed vaccination drive didn't even have the fringe benefit of protecting locals against hepatitis: the second shot of the vaccine, required for immunity, was never given. But when the story of the operation leaked, it stoked suspicions in Pakistan that all vaccination campaigns were part of a Western plot. The Taliban took aim at polio vaccination workers in both Afghanistan and Pakistan, and ever more parents refused to have their children immunized. In 2014, the White House announced that it was no longer CIA policy to make operational use of vaccination programs, but the damage had been done.

Even among the great majority worldwide who believe vaccines are safe, many fail to act. Most vaccinations are given as an automatic part of pediatrician visits. But when they aren't, vaccination rates drop dramatically. In 2012, if the influenza vaccine rate had hit 70 percent rather than the actual level of 45 percent, thirty thousand fewer people would have been hospitalized in the US with flu. Some may have had the excuse that it was too difficult or expensive to get the shot, perhaps others were ignorant of the benefits, but for too many (including me, I'm ashamed to say) the only explanation is they were too selfish or lazy to avail themselves of protection—despite the benefits that provides for others.

Alongside under-use of proven sanitation and vaccination techniques, *overuse* of some of our weapons against infection is also a risk. A comparatively minor concern with overuse is that disinfecting wipes and HEPA filters may be driving our infection-fighting cells to distraction. If not exposed to enough microbes early in life, the immune system may start fighting against the wrong thing—developing allergies as a reaction against pollen, for example. It can sound counterintuitive—or at the very least, like bad parenting—but setting babies down on the rug and giving them a bit of exposure to bacteria carried on cockroaches, mice, and cat dander may make them less likely to develop asthma later on.[27] Conversely, exposing children to triclosan—the active ingredient in antibacterial soap—may increase the likelihood they'll be diagnosed with allergies or hay fever.[28] There's some evidence that early exposure to antibiotics leads to obesity as well.[29] That isn't to say we were better off in the age of mass infection. Allergies are a good deal better than a case of cholera. But exposure to at least some minor infection risks may be better than no exposure at all.

The more serious examples of overuse involve taking our sharpest weapons against infection and blunting them through profligate deployment, increasing the risk of a return to higher rates of disease. And that's linked to the evolution of both microbes and the vector animals that carry them, most significantly mosquitoes. Overuse puts a time limit on the efficiency of a range of different infection-fighting tools, something we've been battling for more than a half century.

In 1958, President Eisenhower used his State of the Union address to declare war on an infectious disease: "We now have it within our power to eradicate from the face of the earth that age-old scourge of mankind: malaria. We are embarking with other nations in an all-out five-year campaign to blot out this curse forever," he announced.[30]

The miracle that would allow America to achieve this goal was a pesticide: dichloro-diphenyl-trichloroethane. DDT spraying was intended to kill mosquitoes, while the drug chloroquine (an artificial relative of quinine from the fever tree) was used to suppress the malaria parasites in infected people. The combined approach had worked to almost completely wipe out the problem of US soldiers succumbing to malaria as they fought across the Pacific in the Second World War.

Sadly, DDT wasn't only used to spray houses during the global malaria campaign—it was widely used on crops to increase yields by killing bugs that ate plants. That helped speed the evolution of DDT-resistant mosquitoes. (It also meant that the chemical entered the environmental food chain: in the US that decimated populations of animals including the peregrine falcon.) Not for the last time, as we'll see, a potentially powerful weapon for human health was blunted by inappropriate use in agriculture. And owing in part to incomplete treatments and poor quality drugs, the malaria parasite evolved as well, developing resistance to the anti-malarial drug chloroquine.[31] In some parts of the world, malaria rebounded to kill more than ever.[32] Soon after, the US, the major backer for global eradication efforts, pulled funding.

Around one-half of the world's countries have eliminated malaria, most in the period after the Second World War. Of the ninety-nine still blighted by the disease, thirty-two are pursuing an elimination strategy, including China, Mexico, Argentina, and South Africa.[33]

There is still hope that humanity can eradicate the disease.[34] That points to the importance of newer techniques to reduce mosquito populations, including genetic manipulation of the insects.

And the eradication effort will have to respond to growing resistance not just to chloroquine but also to an alternative treatment, artemisinin, spreading from the Mekong Delta where it first emerged. The planet has seen dramatic progress against malaria in the last decade, but that means there are more and more young people unexposed. If they stop sleeping under bed nets, or if spraying is reduced or becomes less effective, the disease could roar back as it has before.[35]

It isn't just malaria that is showing stubborn resistance to drugs: in Europe and America HIV that is resistant to at least one antiretroviral drug infects between 10 and 17 percent of patients, even if they haven't used antiretrovirals previously.[36] Multidrug-resistant tuberculosis is also spreading—the result of people failing to complete their treatment because of irregular supply or lack of medical supervision.[37] Curing one patient of extensively drug-resistant tuberculosis costs as much as treating two hundred patients with nonresistant tuberculosis.[38] But perhaps the biggest concern with resistance involves general-use antibiotics, where a return to a pre-antibiotic world would be catastrophic for modern medicine.

Antibiotic resistance has been around almost as long as the drugs themselves. Alexander Fleming himself understood the dangers of antibiotics misuse—in his acceptance speech for the Nobel Prize in Medicine in 1945 he warned that "it is not difficult to make microbes resistant to penicillin in the laboratory by exposing them to concentrations not sufficient to kill them."[39]

And it did not take long for resistant microbes to start killing people. In 1972, an outbreak of typhoid fever exploded in Mexico, infecting more than ten thousand people. The condition leaves victims feeling weak, with stomach pains and headaches, and fevers reaching 104 degrees. Untreated, as many as 20 percent of sufferers can die.[40] The *Salmonella typhi* bacterium can be killed with antibiotics. Doctors in Mexico prescribed chloramphenicol—a powerful antimicrobial that usually drops mortality rates well below 1 percent. But the treatment didn't work. The bacteria simply wouldn't die. Worse, a range of other antibiotics also proved ineffective, including streptomycin, sulfonamide, and tetracycline. Antibiotic-resistant *Salmonella typhi* were found in the early 1970s in countries as far apart as Singapore, India, and the United Kingdom.

E. S. Anderson of the United Kingdom's Enteric Reference Laboratory, who tracked the spread of the resistant bacteria, explained what was behind it:

> The cause of the rise of chloramphenicol resistance in the typhoid bacillus is unfortunately only too evident. It is the result of the widespread, protracted and indiscriminate use of chloramphenicol and other antibiotics in man and animals.[41]

Every time an antibiotic is prescribed, there is a risk that resistance to that antibiotic will develop: some bacteria may survive the treatment because of a greater genetic tolerance. If they go on to infect again, once again the bacteria that are naturally more resistant to antibiotics will be more likely to thrive. The more antibiotics are used, the more opportunity there is for resistance to develop. And the risk is magnified if patients don't finish their course of antibiotics or use low doses or substandard drugs—because more bacteria will survive.

That makes profligate prescription a deadly problem. Half of all the antibiotics that are prescribed to people in the US aren't needed or aren't optimally effective. For example, only 10 percent of acute bronchitis cases in the US are caused by bacteria, but doctors prescribe antibiotics to treat the condition 70 percent of the time.[42] You can even buy antibiotics online without a prescription—a recent study found 136 sellers would ship them to the US, for example, which means many people buy them direct for illnesses for which they'll be of no help.[43] And the US is hardly the worst case.[44] The average person in China consumes ten times the volume of antibiotics each year as a person in America. Worldwide, around half of all antibiotics for human use are purchased from private vendors without a prescription.[45]

The resistance problem is exacerbated by the antibiotic dosing that is occurring with animals—indeed, most antibiotics don't go to treat people but are used on farms. In the 1940s, researchers accidentally discovered that giving livestock feed laced with antibiotics could make them grow faster. Subsequently, farmers began routinely administering small doses of antibiotics to their hogs, cattle, and chicken. In the US today, four-fifths of antibiotics produced each year are used in agriculture, largely to enhance growth. By making this dosing routine—especially on factory farms—we've taken a historically significant source of new human infections, supersized it, and given the infections a perfect environment to develop immunity to our most powerful tools to fight them. The result is unsurprising.

In 1976, microbiologist Dr. Stuart B. Levy traveled forty miles to the west of Boston and set up a farm with 300 chickens. The birds were separated into two groups—one set of 150 birds was given normal feed while the other was fed grain laced with the antibiotic oxytetracycline. The research team collected bird droppings from each group and tested them in the lab. Within two days of the experiment's start the birds fed the antibiotic were excreting out E. coli bacteria that were resistant to stronger doses of tetracycline. And after three months on the feed, the chickens were excreting E. coli that wasn't just resistant to the antibiotic that they'd been fed but a range of others: sulfonamide, ampicillin, streptomycin, and carbenicillin.

Levy's team also examined the feces of the family working the farm. The E. coli that had worked its way through their intestines was *also* resistant to multiple antibiotics, far more than that of farmers on neighboring properties who weren't using antibiotic-laced feed. Farmworkers had been exposed by breathing in aerosolized chicken feces. Most E. coli are harmless to humans, but some strains cause diarrhea, urinary tract infections, respiratory illnesses, and pneumonia, among other conditions. The study demonstrated that low-dosage antibiotic use on farms increased the risk of antibiotic-resistant infections spreading to humans.

Four decades after Dr. Levy's experiment, the microbiologist testified to the US House Committee on Energy and Commerce. He reported that, despite considerable additional research on the problem, "we are not gaining ground in the struggle against antibiotic resistance and all of us—you, me, and your constituents—are at ever greater risk of contracting a resistant bacterial infection and even one that is untreatable."[46]

That is because, for all Stuart Levy's work and warnings, we're still using the same drugs to dose animals as we use to protect people against septic cuts, or heal from surgery, or recover from a stomach bug. Nearly two-thirds of the drugs used in animal feed in the US—20 million pounds of antibiotics a year—are medically important for use in people.[47] And China may consume as much as two hundred thousand metric tons of antibiotics each year, ten times US consumption.[48]

US government tests of meat sold in supermarkets suggest that 50 percent of chicken samples contain campylobacter bacteria that is resistant to the antibiotic tetracyclin; moreover, of the salmonella found in chicken samples, half of it is multidrug-resistant.[49] Campylobacter causes a week-long case of diarrhea often accompanied by vomiting, while salmonella infection is also associated with diarrhea, along with fever and abdominal cramps.[50]

And in November 2015, Chinese scientists found, in both pigs and humans, mutant bacteria, including E. coli, that was resistant to all available antibiotics.[51] If and when total resistance spreads in a more harmful microbe, doctors and patients will be faced with an infection for which they can do very little.

With 1 billion plus pigs farmed worldwide, many fed a diet of low-dose antibiotics to aid growth, others fed with a cannibal diet of pig offal, we've created a global porcine petri dish for developing new superbugs. Bacon may be a crispy and delicious part of breakfast, but it can also be a crispy and delicious infectious disease–breeding nemesis if we don't rein in inappropriate antibiotic use.

Resistant microbes that cause infections of the urinary tract and bloodstream, pneumonia, septic wounds, meningitis, and diarrhea are expanding planet-wide.[52] Infection's most famous mass killer, bubonic plague, has evolved an antibiotic-resistant strain.[53] And the Centers for Disease Control suggests that fifteen infections are urgent or serious threats in that they're resistant to multiple antibiotics, including drug-resistant tuberculosis and methicillin-resistant *Staphylococcus aureus* (MRSA, which causes skin abscesses filled with bacteria that can burrow toward bones and lungs).

We lack accurate data on the scale of deaths related to antibiotic resistance. An investigation by journalists Ryan McNeill, Deborah Nelson, and Yasmeen Abutaleb found widespread underreporting of antibiotic-resistant conditions on death certificates even in the US. For example, Emma Grace Breaux was reported to have died of pneumonia at age three, but unmentioned on the certificate was that her heart and lungs had been severely weakened by a case of MRSA she contracted at the hospital where she was born. Joshua Nahum was preparing to go home after a month in the hospital after a skydiving accident, but contracted drug-resistant bacteria that caused sufficient brain swelling to kill him. The death certificate blandly listed "delayed complications" from his injuries. Few states require notification of drug-resistant outbreaks in hospitals, and the hospitals themselves have little incentive to report what is in part the result of insufficient attention to sanitation by their staff.[54]

But the best estimates are that MRSA kills eighteen thousand people a year in the United States alone.[55] The toll in Europe and the US from antimicrobial resistance as a whole is around fifty thousand a year.[56] Worldwide, resistant bacteria already kill as many as seven hundred thousand people a year—seven times the mortality burden of cholera and six times that of measles.[57] And resistance is a problem that has the risk of exploding.

There are many ways the post-antibiotic era would be a catastrophe—not least, it could bring surgery back toward the nineteenth century. In 2013, Tom Frieden, at that point US Centers for Disease Control director, warned:

> Losing effective treatment will not only undermine our ability to fight routine infections, but also have serious complications, serious implications, for people who have other medical problems. For example, things like joint replacements and organ transplants, cancer chemotherapy and diabetes treatment, treatment of rheumatoid arthritis. All of these are dependent on our ability to fight infections that may be exacerbated by the treatment of these conditions. And if we lose our antibiotics, we'll lose the ability to do that effectively.[58]

Despite surgeons vowing to clean their hands, arms, and instruments with (even greater) care, the risk of postoperative infection would multiply. And every surgical procedure would become dramatically more dangerous. If antibiotics don't work on an infected wound, for example, surgeons are forced to use the state-of-the-art treatment that prevailed in the 1930s: debridement. That involves trying to cut out all of the infected tissue and is more dangerous and far more invasive than a course of penicillin.[59] As we overprescribe antibiotics, creating a range of antibiotic-resistant superbugs, we may speedily regress toward a world in which maggots (that eat putrefying flesh) become our best defense against gangrene. Indeed, they're *already* commercially available for the treatment of wounds responding poorly to antibiotics.[60]

A review of the antimicrobial threat, sponsored by the British government and chaired by economist Jim O'Neill, predicts that, by 2050, 10 million people could be dying a year from increased antimicrobial resistance worldwide if we fail to act. That's more than die worldwide each year from cancer. It compares to a World Health Organization estimate of 250,000 additional deaths each year from the effects of climate change between 2030 and 2050.[61] Global deaths from terrorism run at about one one-thousandth of the potential toll of antibiotic resistance.[62] (Compare the attention paid by newspapers, cable news, or presidential debates to the three issues: terror comes first and climate second, with antibiotics finishing a distant third.)

Meanwhile, the number of new drug approvals for antibacterials has been dropping, while the gap between antibiotic introduction and the emergence of resistant infections appears to be shrinking. It took nine years between the introduction of the antibiotic tetracycline and the identification of tetracycline-resistant shigella. It took one year between the introduction of ceftaroline and the identification of ceftaroline-resistant staphylococcus.[63] Our profligacy with use increases research costs to find new alternatives, and in the meantime treatment costs tick steadily upward. But we're doing little to increase research budgets for new drugs.

Making matters worse is the ongoing military research aimed at making infection threats more deadly so that they can be weaponized.

Humans have abused the power of parasites in war for a long time. An ancient torture described by Plutarch used maggots' taste for the distasteful to slowly consume a victim encased between two boats.[64] We've seen early accounts of Tartars catapulting the corpses of Black Death victims into the besieged town of Caffa. And the Venetian doctor Michiel Angelo Salamon tried a more complex variation of the same approach. He distilled liquids collected from the spleen, buboes, and carbuncles of plague-stricken victims as a potential bioweapon.[65]

A more effective historical attempt at biological warfare involved British colonists giving Native Americans blankets dusted in smallpox scabs. It was an approach that General Washington feared the British would turn on his troops as they marched on Boston, and it led him to order the entire army inoculated through the process of variolation.[66]

Microbes were, of course, also used as weapons of war in the twentieth century. Jiang Chun Geng is a farmer who lives in Dachen, China. He was born in 1930 and was caught up in the brutal war between Japan and his country at the age of twelve. His whole family became infected with festering sores soon after Japanese soldiers passed through his village, as he reported to Judith Miller of the Manhattan Institute. His mother and younger brother died from the sores. But he lived on, with a decomposing and swollen right leg that, sixty years later, remained a putrid open wound.[67]

As reported by Miller, Jiang was the victim of biological warfare, carried out by the euphemistically titled Epidemic Prevention and Water Purification Department—Unit 731 of the Imperial Japanese Army. Over the period 1932 to 1945, the unit performed experiments on prisoners of war that involved intentional infection and investigative surgery. As well, it carried out germ warfare involving plague, anthrax, and typhus. Around the Chinese city of Harbin, soldiers laced one thousand wells with typhoid bacilli and handed out bottles of lemonade injected with typhus to local children. In Nanking, they distributed anthrax-filled chocolate and cake to kids. They even took their experiments far enough to discover new vectors: a US Army report on the unit's accomplishments notes "one of the greatest" was the use of the human flea to infect victims with the plague in the Chinese city of Changteh—showing you didn't need rats to spread the Black Death.[68]

But Unit 731 also followed a more traditional route by mixing fleas infected with the bacteria into bags of rice and wheat, which they dropped over the city of Quzhou in October 1940. The rats ate the grain and picked up the plague-carrying fleas. For whatever reason, *Yersinia pestis* had lost its edge since the Black Death—perhaps sanitary conditions were better in wartime China than they'd been in Europe of the Middle Ages. Only 121 people died of the resulting plague outbreak.[69]

US General Douglas MacArthur recognized cutting-edge innovation when he saw it. The perpetrators never faced war crimes charges, with most of the research team co-opted into the US biowarfare program in exchange for immunity. Jiang, along with other victims, has never received reparations for what was done to him, and the Japanese government still refuses to acknowledge the program, which may have killed many thousands in attacks across seventy towns and cities.

More recently, in 2001, letters laced with anthrax spores were sent to US senators and media outlets, along with notes saying what the spores were and that the recipient might want to visit a hospital. The letters clearly weren't designed to maximize death, but they did demonstrate the risk of biological weapons, as well as the ease of hiding their production—no one has been charged in connection with the crime. The airborne release of one kilogram of anthrax aerosol over New York could kill hundreds of thousands—and anthrax that is antibiotic-resistant has been developed by both the US and the former Soviet Union.[70]

In 2003, then US secretary of state Colin Powell presented evidence to the UN Security Council regarding Iraq's weapons of mass destruction and used the anthrax incident as an example. At one point he picked up a vial of liquid and noted, "Less than a teaspoon of dry anthrax . . . in an envelope shut down the United States Senate in the fall of 2001." Saddam Hussein could have produced twenty-five thousand liters of anthrax, he confided. "We have first-hand descriptions of biological weapons factories on wheels and on rails. . . . They can produce anthrax and botulinum toxin. In fact, they can produce enough dry biological agent in a single month to kill thousands upon thousands of people."[71]

As we now know, while Iraq previously had a bioweapons program, the anthrax was either never made or was destroyed prior to the US invasion. But biological warfare remains a real risk. Indeed, in the future, it's possible that the biggest threat to the vast majority of humanity from infectious disease will be a bioengineered weapon of mass destruction.

Compared to building an atomic weapon—which involves a nuclear power plant or complex enrichment infrastructure alongside advanced engineering and conventional explosives technology—bioweapons are straightforward to manufacture. The Manhattan Project to develop the atom bomb in World War Two was comparable in manpower and capital cost to the entire prewar automobile industry of the United States. Today, single university labs regularly create bioweapons, sometimes by accident. According to Nathan Myhrvold, former chief technology officer for Microsoft, the technology of molecular biology manipulation means that "access to mass death has been democratized; it has spread from a small elite of superpower leaders to nearly anybody with modest resources." Indeed, a team of virologists at the University of Wisconsin-Madison has listed the simple changes they would need to make to convert a lethal strain of bird flu into something that could be easily transmitted between mammals.

The small individual scale of operations is why the Soviet Union could secretly continue a massive bioweapons program after a 1972 treaty with the US banned their production. More alarming even than the ease with which these killer pathogens can be produced is that, in contrast to a single nuclear dirty bomb that spreads radioactive material or even a Hiroshima-sized nuclear weapon, the right biological agent can spread worldwide, killing on every continent.[72] And the international treaty meant to prevent states from working on infectious threats, the Biological Weapons Convention, lacks significant verification mechanisms, leaving the world at the mercy of the goodwill of its signatories.

But once again, the threat comes not only from the risk but, also, our response to it. The recent history of bioterror suggests significant limits to terrorists' practical ability to create effective weapons: the 1984 tainting of salad with salmonella in Oregon by the Rajneeshee religious cult killed no one; the 2001 anthrax mailings killed very few.[73] And Colin Powell's UN speech was part of an effort to justify the invasion of Iraq on what turned out to be faulty grounds.

Just as naturally occurring infectious disease has often been used as an excuse to deny liberties, the risk of bioterror was one justification for the growth of fortress America—including increased military spending, greater use of targeted assassination, torture, invasive intelligence-gathering operations, and complex, expensive visa and screening requirements for visitors to the US. It's not clear that, on net, these programs make Americans safer (let alone the world).[74] They certainly have considerable spillover effects—including reduced effectiveness in fighting infectious disease itself, as we've seen in the case of polio eradication.

There are many diseases we're unlikely to wipe out for a long time if ever: infections such as Covid-19, Ebola, and plague that have animal reservoirs, as well as conditions like flu that mutate so fast and spread so rapidly that we're constantly playing catch-up. And new diseases will continue to emerge—hopefully, only from nature, but perhaps including man-made threats. As long as we remain a planet of 7-plus billion, close-packed and widely traveled, with a love for meat, eggs, and milk, infections will be a force in our lives.

The only question is "How big?" We have the technology and resources to confine infection to the status of a minor global annoyance—killing few, temporarily disabling more, but in the bush leagues of death rates. But there is also the pessimistic view: we have the technology—and infections have the natural capacity—to become a massive force for global death and decline. And we can make the future even darker by reacting late and at a cost to liberties. The choice is ours.

CHAPTER ELEVEN

Flattening the Plague Cycle

By 2030, end preventable deaths of newborns and children under 5 years of age . . .

—United Nations Sustainable Development Goals

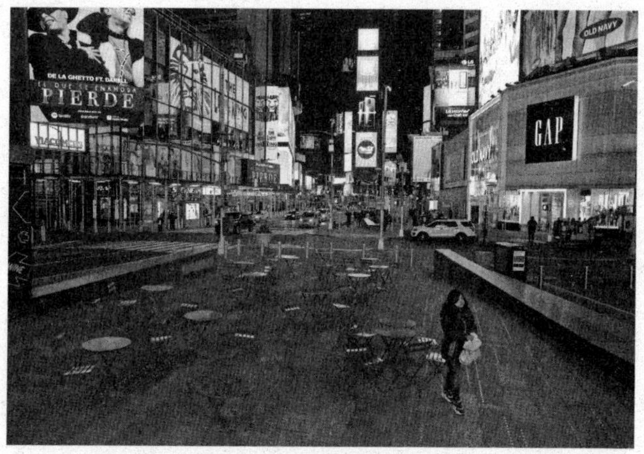

Covid-19 lockdown empties Times Square.
(Source: AP Photo/Seth Wenig)

The fight against infection is a public fight. Individuals acting alone can only do so much to counter it. That's why responses to the infectious disease threat have involved ever growing government involvement. In 1868, Sir John Simon, medical officer of health for the City of London, proudly enumerated the extended powers of government that had already developed to respond to disease in Victorian Britain. The state

> "has interfered between parent and child, not only in imposing limitation on industrial uses of children, but also to the extent of requiring children should not be left unvaccinated. It has interfered between employer and employed [insisting] certain sanitary claims shall be fulfilled . . . between vendor and purchaser . . . and has made it a public offense to sell adulterated food or drink or medicine. . . . It has provided that in any sort of epidemic emergency organized medical assistance, not peculiarly for paupers, may be required of local authorities."[1]

Dorothy Porter suggests that public health interventions were viewed by early Victorians as "the most infamous growth of authoritarian, paternalist power of central government . . . and the growth of the despotic influence of a particular profession—the medical profession."[2] Nonetheless, the authoritarians, paternalists, and despots won. Since then the (necessary) intrusions have only grown.

But there's still more to be done. In 2017, about 10 million people died from communicable diseases worldwide. Many of those deaths were preventable. We need to extend the full benefits of the sanitation and medical revolution. And we need to improve our response to new disease threats. Both efforts will necessarily be *global.* Just as no one individual or family can fully respond to the infectious threat, in a globalized world neither can any one country.

Even though everyone is at threat from infection, it's among poor people in poor countries where that threat most often translates into dying. That's because while fighting infectious disease is cheaper than dealing with the diseases of the rich, poor countries have incomes so low that even simple preventatives are out of reach.

Take the response to HIV: we have seen that for the first time in 2013, more people worldwide were put on antiretrovirals than were newly infected from the disease.[3] And costs for those antiretroviral drugs had come down markedly. That price decline was delayed by the monopoly (patent) rights given to companies that develop new drugs. But even after generic (off-patent) producers entered the market, antiretrovirals remained a very expensive way to save lives in Africa: their cost of about $350 per year of life saved compared to $42 per life year for programs that support adult male circumcision (which reduces HIV transmission), $24 or less per life year for extending bed net coverage against malaria, and $5 or less per life year for increasing vaccination coverage.[4]

The average annual health expenditure in the world's poorest countries is just $10 per person—about half of that private expenditure and about half from the government. (In the US, health dollars spent are closer to $6,000 per person per year.) If you were a minister of health responsible for a budget that could amount to as little as $5 per person in your population, and the list of needs included everything from shots to cancer treatments, how would you spend the money: on comparatively expensive treatments to keep AIDS patients alive or, rather, on bed nets that would save more people for the same price? In a world that's as rich as ours, no one should be forced to make decisions like that.

In 2013, the Lancet Global Health Commission, chaired by former treasury secretary Lawrence Summers, declared that the world can and should provide universal access to a range of cheap and effective global health services, most focused on infectious diseases, by 2035. These would prevent about 15 million deaths a year in the world's poorest eighty-two countries, those classified as low-income or lower-middle-income by the World Bank. The commission estimated that most countries could afford to finance these interventions by themselves, but the poorest countries as a group might require a total of $9 billion in aid financing. That is approximately one-fifteenth of current global aid flows, suggesting it's eminently affordable.

Admittedly, a greater challenge may be ensuring that the money committed is turned into improved outcomes in countries where a lot of care is distinctly substandard.[5] A recent World Bank–sponsored survey of practice in Nigerian health clinics and hospitals tested to see if doctors and nurses followed clinical guidelines in asking basic questions when presented with patients complaining of symptoms of common illnesses, if they diagnosed the illnesses correctly, and if basic medical tools and basic drugs were available to treat such conditions. The survey indicated a national average of 32 percent adherence to clinical guidelines, 36 percent diagnostic accuracy, and 44 percent drug availability. Slightly more than two-thirds of facilities did at least have one working thermometer.

Nigeria is hardly the exception in Sub-Saharan Africa, and national averages hide even worse outcomes in rural hospitals.[6]

Frustratingly, donors in rich countries have to date focused on particular disease campaigns—including against malaria, polio, and AIDS—almost to the exclusion of supporting the development of functioning health systems. For all of the great success against smallpox and polio and the significant progress against malaria and AIDS, health improvements will only continue if broader health networks work.[7] They deserve more support.

Beyond the health sector, the more that basic sanitation systems function, the less people will need treatments and cures in the first place. The World Bank estimates that it would cost $28 billion a year between now and 2030 to reach universal global access to basic water, sanitation, and hygiene facilities. That means clean water less than fifteen minutes' walk away and at least a decent pit-latrine to use as a toilet. Making sure that every household has its *own* clean water supply, and a toilet that can safely dispose of feces, would cost $114 billion a year.[8]

That's a lot of money (and, again, it will take more than money). On the other hand, given the global burden of disease related to poor sanitation, it might seem like a bargain.

It may be that technology can come to the rescue, lowering costs. The Gates Foundation is backing the development of toilets that will need no water or sewage to convert urine and feces into pathogen-free manure or electrical energy—at a cost below 5 cents per user per day.[9] A number of different models are being piloted in developing countries—if they work, they'd hugely simplify the provision of sanitation and could dramatically reduce the risk of feces-related infection in slums and cities worldwide.

Achieving further dramatic global reductions in infection will also take behavior change: doctors correctly diagnosing and treating, nurses turning up to work, but, most important, people using basic sanitary techniques. Once again, we have some idea how that is done: in 2001, the Indian government launched the Total Sanitation Campaign. Learning from earlier efforts in which latrines were constructed only for them to sit unused or be converted into storage sheds, the government put a lot of effort into fostering use. In some areas, village leaders were given a cash bonus if their village was declared open defecation–free. The program was a partial success—open defecation dropped from 64 to 53 percent of households over the period from 2001 to 2011. And fully eliminating open-field defecation in a village had a dramatic impact on child heights—significantly reducing stunting.[10] But that it took ten years of effort to reduce open defecation by one-sixth demonstrates how hard it can be to make progress.

The world's governments also need to work together to eradicate some of the worst infectious threats, including polio, measles, and malaria. Such efforts are some of the highest-return investments we can make. The eradication of smallpox, beyond saving somewhere over 40 million lives worldwide since the 1970s,[11] also avoided $2 billion a year in vaccination and hospital expenditures in the US alone—an impressive return for a global program that only cost around $300 million, and for a disease that had already been almost completely eliminated as a domestic health threat in the US before the global eradication program began.[12] The US recoups its investment in the global smallpox eradication effort once every twenty-six days.[13]

When it comes to protecting some of our most valuable tools in the fight against infection, much depends on a new set of global agreements around drug quality and antibiotic use. Take antibiotic use in animals: the economic case for truly global action is urgent and overwhelming. That's not least because the benefits of antibiotic use in agriculture have proved limited: antibiotics substitute for improved farm sanitation in a way that is, at best, marginally effective. Economic analysis suggests that the slightly slower growth of pigs taken off antibiotics might raise farm-gate meat prices by perhaps 1 percent.[14] Meanwhile, the harmful impact of livestock-related resistance is both considerable and global.

An international agreement on antibiotic use in animals could, as a first phase, mandate the rapid reduction of the use of antimicrobials also used in humans, followed by phase-out of all antibiotic use for growth promotion, with support for farmers in poorer countries to encourage heightened use of sanitary techniques and other alternatives. Perhaps there could be similar agreements aimed at phasing out multi-use needles, or tightening requirements for human antibiotic use.

The world's governments should also come together to fund research toward new vaccines, antimicrobials, and vector control. A particular problem with respect to drug development is that a market that focuses on current diseases of the rich denies the world cures to diseases that mostly affect the poor. Case in point: we have multiple cures for erectile dysfunction but lack a single malaria vaccine.[15]

The total global market for all vaccines is about two-thirds of the market for the single cholesterol-reducing drug Lipitor.[16] The antibiotics market, though also vital to health, is similarly unrewarding. This is a matter of rich-world self-interest: if we want to reduce the risk of a global breakout by a disease customarily found in a developing country, the best response is proactive research and development, and that's going to take global cooperation.

One response to the research problem was developed in 2009 by the Gavi Alliance—a consortium of donors that support vaccine purchases for the world's poorest countries. The alliance wanted to spur the creation of a vaccine to fight pneumococcal strains in developing countries—a bacteria that causes pneumonia, meningitis, and sepsis. Pneumococcal diseases killed 1.6 million people each year in poorer countries, accounting for one out of every four child deaths.[17] Instead of funding research and development, the Alliance simply guaranteed that they'd spend $1.5 billion to buy the vaccine at $7 per dose if drug companies manufactured it.

Drug companies rose to the challenge. Only two years later, GlaxoSmithKline and Pfizer had rolled out suitable products, and a number of developing country drug manufacturers were close behind.

Besides increasing research funding, we should be rushing out similar commitments for new antibiotics or vaccines for diseases like malaria. The new Center for Epidemic Preparedness Innovations, backed by donors including the governments of Norway and Japan, is supporting research, development, regulatory trials, and stockpiling of vaccines for potential outbreak diseases including Lassa fever, Nipah, MERS, and Ebola (it's also supporting work on a Covid-19 vaccine).[18]

Other approaches include manipulating mosquito DNA so that mosquitoes are incapable of carrying malaria, and using "gene drive" technology to ensure that nearly all offspring develop the desired traits. Drastically reducing the global population of mosquitoes—or, at least, reducing them to a nuisance rather than the world's most deadly animal—would be a massive boon.

Controlling the risk of new infectious outbreaks and pandemics is first and foremost about getting public health systems to work. Take Ebola: for it to spread, the bodily fluids of an infected person need direct contact with an open wound or the mucous membranes of another. We've seen that despite its lethality, it's an unlikely candidate to spark a global pandemic when the natural response through the ages—staying away from people who look sick—is such a powerful preventative.

It is a sign of the weakness of health systems in parts of West Africa that Ebola spread at all in 2014. In that year, Nigeria saw nine laboratory-confirmed cases of the disease, and patients were rapidly isolated. Health authorities followed up with nearly nine hundred patient contacts and kept the contacts under observation for twenty-one days. The disease was stopped in its tracks.[19] Nigeria has an income per capita that is one-tenth the level in the US—showing that even poor developing countries can control the condition.

The same is broadly true of *all* infectious diseases: if you can find and isolate patients and sterilize contact, the chain of infection should be broken. It is in everyone's interest that every country can provide at least the bare minimum of health coverage and epidemic preparedness to support that response for less contagious conditions such as Ebola.

We learned in 2020 that the challenge is considerably greater with a disease that can spread so easily from people who are showing few if any symptoms. That said, we've known most of the effective responses to a contagious pandemic for a hundred years or more by now. US cities and states responded to the 1918 flu by issuing public service announcements about risk and by increasing hospital surge capacity; closures, quarantines, and social distancing measures; disease surveillance; and vaccine research and distribution.[20] The problem both in 1918 and 102 years after wasn't that we didn't know what to do, it was that many countries didn't do it well.

In the early stages of the Covid-19 response, many countries, including the US, failed to properly communicate: leaders underplayed the risk the virus presented as well as the response that would be required; they led through bad example when it came to enforcing social distancing and wearing masks; and they touted treatments that had no scientific basis. Hospitals struggled to deal with the patient load and reported a lack of isolation units, ventilators, and supplies of basic protective equipment including masks. Social distancing measures were introduced too late in many regions and removed too soon in others; and it took far too long to ramp up capacity to test, trace contacts, and isolate the infected.

Meanwhile, other countries achieved early victories against the disease. South Korea, scarred by a poor performance battling the Middle East respiratory syndrome outbreak in 2015, had considerably bolstered its capacity to respond. By early March 2020, it had tested more people for Covid-19 than the US, the UK, France, Italy, and Japan combined. It also imposed strict isolation of sick people in hospitals and dorms—away from families or group houses. In mid-March, the US and South Korea each had about ninety Covid-19 fatalities. During the month of April, South Korea lost eighty-five more people to the disease while the US lost sixty-two thousand.[21]

Still, worldwide, attempts to limit the coronavirus's spread by reducing contact were unprecedented in scale—a far broader shutdown than achieved by Italian cities confronting the plague seven centuries ago, and more widespread and longer-lasting than the school shutdowns, prohibitions on public gatherings, and quarantines put in place by US cities during the 1918 influenza pandemic.[22]

We've seen that because of their (appropriately) impressive scale, these efforts carried immense cost. That cost could have been reduced, and, more important, lives could have been saved, if countries had been better prepared. For future outbreaks, governments should expand their stockpiles of masks, basic medical equipment, and drugs. And given that countries that tested many of their citizens early have seen fewer cases and less disruption, every nation should be creating the infrastructure and gathering the equipment to roll out testing, tracing, and isolation.

From their experiences with Covid-19 governments should also learn what level of isolation is sustainable and for how long. During the 1918 flu pandemic, distancing measures helped slow spread, but they didn't have a significant effect on overall death rates.[23] In part, that may be because they were abandoned too soon. Realistically, there is no one-size-fits-all solution to what is a sustainable level of shutdown and social distancing—and that suggests the need for individual planning by governments worldwide.

One thing that determines how long and how much people can remain distanced is how long they can *afford* to do so. For some lucky, largely better off employees, working from home is straightforward. For others, work necessitates going somewhere else. Many of the biggest coronavirus hot spots in the US were large workplaces, including meat packing plants, aircraft carriers, and nursing homes. Providing financial support to ensure those who don't need to go to work don't have to, and providing protective equipment and training to the rest, is a tool both to reduce the economic impact of infection and to save lives. The programs started in 2020 in countries including Brazil, the UK, and the US to extend unemployment benefits, provide universal income support, or pay employers to retain workers were all steps in that direction. Thinking through financial mechanisms to equitably cushion the cost of lockdowns is a vital part of pandemic preparation.

Another lesson we learned again from Covid-19 is how much we need improved planetary cooperation to confront pandemics. Ever since we've had a global disease pool, we've needed global responses to deal with it. Slowly, too slowly, we've built some of that capacity. In fact, some of the earliest cooperative international agreements involved pandemic response: in the 1830s, there was a treaty on quarantine in the Mediterranean, for example. The International Cholera Control Commission met in Istanbul in 1866 to impose a quarantine against ships coming from India, much to the disgust of free-trading British ministers.[24] And in 1898, an international conference on the spread of Yunnan plague was held in Venice. Once again, the government of India was chided for its lack of action on the disease and quarantines were imposed on Indian exports.[25]

More recently, under the auspices of the World Health Organization, there's been global cooperation to track and combat infection. And the response to outbreaks including swine flu and bird flu has shown that the web of international treaties, however threadbare, can still achieve results. The International Health Regulations obligate countries to notify the World Health Organization within twenty-four hours of any event that may constitute a "public health emergency of international concern"—and with the 2009 swine flu outbreak that was broadly what happened.

At the same time, the regulations call for improved detection and reporting capacity of health events.[26] But in 2013, out of 193 member countries, the WHO judged that only 80 countries were displaying the core capacities required for hazard alert and response. The World Health Organization itself has limited capacity. Member countries flatlined the institution's core budget beginning in the 1980s. From 1993 onward, the policy has been one of zero nominal growth—with no accounting for inflation. Today, its budget is worth about 30 cents per person per year worldwide.

The WHO's limited capacities were well demonstrated in its response to the West Africa Ebola epidemic. The organization announced the discovery of Ebola in Guinea on March 22, 2014. But in mid-April its spokesman was suggesting "this outbreak isn't different from other outbreaks," which had rapidly petered out. The organization shared a concern with Guinean officials that advertising the potential magnitude of the outbreak could lead to significant economic damage. But it went far too far in accommodating that concern.[27] By the time the emergency was finally announced in early August, 932 people were already dead and there were 1,070 more cases of Ebola.[28]

At that point, if anything, the problem switched to overreaction. The Centers for Disease Control projected that up to 1.4 million could be infected in Liberia and Sierra Leone by January 2015. Global institutions and donor countries rushed late but headlong to respond. Thankfully ignoring nativist calls to quarantine the whole region, governments began mass airlifting of troops and supplies to set up hospitals.

As it turned out, most of those beds were never used. In reality, by January of 2015 there were 19,140 cases—about 1 percent of earlier forecasts.[29] Those are still tragically high numbers for a desperately poor region already suffering an immense disease burden. And they could have been lower if the global response to the outbreak had been early and proportional rather than late and panicked.

The World Health Organization did better in its response to Covid-19. It started daily "situation reports" on Covid on January 21, 2020, when there were only 282 confirmed cases worldwide. By mid-February, the organization was sending Covid-19 laboratory testing kits to member countries, and personal protective equipment to developing countries with the greatest need. At the start of March, it had developed guidance for containment and suppression based on the findings of a joint WHO-China report on the virus and its epidemiology. The guidance was followed by

South Korea and Hong Kong with considerable success. And in March the organization also launched a cross-country "mega-trial" of four potential treatments for Covid-19—big enough to rapidly and accurately demonstrate levels of efficacy.

WHO played an important role in advising against harmful responses, too. Director General Dr. Tedros Adhanom Ghebreyesus warned that all countries "must strike a fine balance between protecting health, minimizing economic and social disruption, and respecting human rights." In the case of Covid-19, the organization advised against the application of travel or trade restrictions for more than short periods.[30]

Many countries didn't fully live up to their commitments under the International Health Regulations. At the year's start, China actively suppressed information on Covid-19 and arrested whistleblowers. It was slow to approve a WHO mission to study the disease. And while WHO advised against travel and trade restrictions, countries including the US ignored that guidance. But, if anything, that suggests the need to *strengthen* the organization.

The International Health Regulations put countries in charge of reporting outbreaks and deny the WHO independent authority to inspect incidents absent host country permission—a significant limit on the organization's ability to monitor infectious threats. When the International Atomic Energy Agency wants to inspect nuclear reactors in a country, it doesn't need to ask nicely and get an invitation first. The Nuclear Nonproliferation Treaty gives the organization authority to verify that the states that have signed on are living up to their obligations not to develop nuclear weapons, and the IAEA's 2,560 staff members are available to carry out those inspections. The same should apply to the World Health Organization in a time of disease outbreaks. (Similarly, more authority and resources should flow to the Implementation Support Unit of the Biological Weapons Convention. The unit needs considerably more than its current four employees, as well as a tighter treaty authority, to conduct investigations around bioweapons production.)[31]

And rather than relying on the capacities of nongovernment groups like Doctors Without Borders and an overstretched WHO core staff to respond to outbreaks, the United Nations should create a body to do for infectious disease what blue-helmeted peacekeeping troops do for war. The WHO's Health Emergencies Program, which leads response to pandemic outbreaks, is chronically underfunded and under capacity. The organization should have access to a roster of volunteers from participating countries who could be called up at short notice to respond to a disease outbreak within days or a few weeks; it should have the ability to call up logistical support from charter companies and (if necessary) the militaries of countries that have agreed to provide transport; finally, it should have access to a significant global stockpile of basic medical supplies.

In April 2020, many of the world's countries were brought together by the World Health Organization to pledge greater cooperation on coronavirus vaccine research and make a commitment to share research, treatment, and medicines globally.[32] That should be the start of a broader effort to create the technological base to better respond to future pandemics. That would include global research in broad-spectrum antivirals and antibiotics that might help fight outbreaks, as well as techniques that allow for more rapid test and vaccine development.

In addition, the world as a whole needs the spare capacity in pharmaceutical manufacturing to quickly scale up vaccine production. Not least, that involves retooling factories in advance of knowing precisely which vaccines will prove effective. In the case of Covid-19, the Gates Foundation supplied some of the funding for this exercise, but the world shouldn't have to rely on private philanthropy to guarantee public health: a dedicated fund under an international organization like the World Health Organization or the World Bank should be able to support rapid development and manufacture of pandemic-response technologies.

Improving global pandemic preparedness wouldn't take a huge amount of money. The Commission on a Global Health Risk Framework for the Future estimates that $4.5 billion a year would buy strengthened national health systems, funding for research and development, and financing to address the most urgent weaknesses in global health security.

Preparing and responding to pandemic threats can't be left in the lap of poorer countries. Not only is it not moral; it isn't *practical.* Ultimately, rapidly spreading infectious disease becomes a problem for all of us wherever it starts, even if the pain is often disproportionately inflicted on poorer regions. We need to ensure that every country has the financial and technical support to confront new threats. That's how the plague has become a minor concern worldwide and how smallpox was eradicated—and it's what the planet needs to achieve with Covid-19 and the pandemics that come after.

The medical and sanitary advances that took place in the twentieth century transformed the world. There's no reason that such advances should stop in the twenty-first. The planet has never been richer—able to afford more research and better disease response. At a cost simply dwarfed by the benefits we can resume our global progress against infection.

CHAPTER TWELVE

Conclusion: Humanity's Greatest Victory

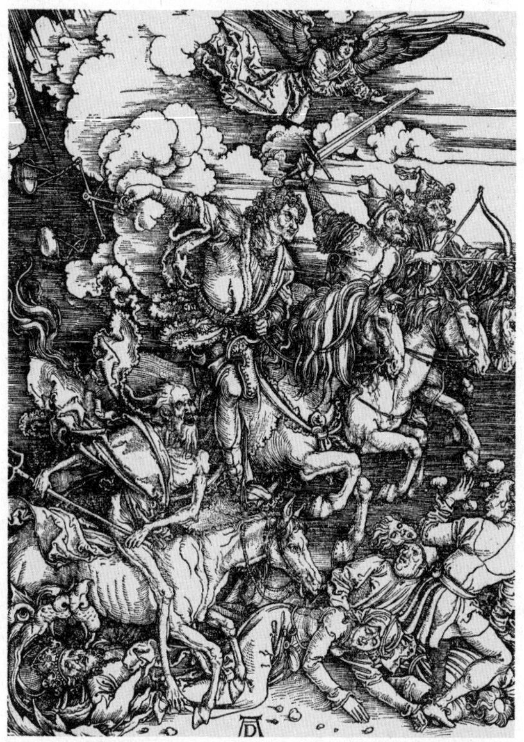

An image from Albrecht Dürer's *The Apocalypse*, featuring the Four Horsemen of the Apocalypse. The rider with the bow is sometimes identified as representing pestilence. (Source: *The Revelation of St. John: The Four Riders of the Apocalypse.* Albrecht Dürer, 1497–98. Wikimedia Commons.)

In the Bible's Book of Revelations, the Four Horsemen of the Apocalypse are sent forth to "kill with sword and with famine and with pestilence and by wild beasts," and carry off a quarter of the earth. The identities of the horsemen are a matter of some debate: the fevered poetry is hard to decipher. While the Fourth Horseman seems to be Death himself, the Third Horseman is universally recognized as famine, and the Second as war, argument rages over the identity of the First Horseman: some recent experts suggest he is pestilence, others argue that he is Jesus Christ or the embodiment of righteousness.

It's ironic that pestilence occupies the disputed saddle, for while throughout most of history violence and famine were two of Death's most useful tools, the only one of the three that has ever managed to carry off a quarter of the earth at one go is pestilence. Plague ended the age of antiquity and ushered in the Renaissance. Infection shaped the age of global empires, and its decline boosted the economy of the modern world. Neither violence nor famine can claim to be its equal.

The frequency of violence, pestilence, and famine combined is why the idea that a good life should be one free of tragedy was mocked as utopian until the Industrial Revolution. They are the tools that nature used to keep humans in Malthusian misery. And none—famine, violence, or pestilence—has nearly the grip on humanity that it had even fifty years ago. A huge part of that progress is due to the fight against infection, flattening the plague cycle, and their knock-on effects.

The extent of disease has always shaped economic and social relations. Pandemics from centuries ago *still* help determine wealth and poverty, democracy and autocracy to this day. But the last half century clearly demonstrates that not all trends are inexorable. We've seen a massive global improvement in the quality of life even in parts of the world that suffered the most from the arrows of the First Horseman through the last two thousand years. Malthusian fatalism had a declining empirical basis in the nineteenth century. Now it has no basis at all.

The tragedy of Covid-19 helps illustrate the utterly different world we've become used to living in. The most alarming early forecasts suggested that if governments and individuals did nothing to respond to the new threat, as many as 2.2 million Americans might die from the coronavirus.[1] That amounts to about six out of every one thousand people in the country. Such forecasts were one factor behind an appropriately massive global response. But in the US in 1900, eight out of every one thousand people died from an infectious disease, and that wasn't an unusual year.[2] For much of human history, it's unlikely that an illness like Covid-19 would have been recognized as a new and distinct health threat at all.

If we continue on the path away from Malthusian doom, which we know how to do, how will the world appear different? With declining birth rates and longer lives, it will undoubtedly be older—but the changes go beyond that. Given the links between infection risk and xenophobia born in prehistory, a less infectious world will be friendlier, more cooperative, and less violent. And given the close link between the rise of infection and the subjugation of women at the dawn of civilization, perhaps it will be more equal. If the pandemic tragedies on the scale of Justinian's plague, the Black Death, and the Atlantic disease exchange go unrepeated, it will be more stable. As good health boosts productivity, countries will be richer and more urbanized—and the gap between industrial and developing countries should continue to shrink. It won't be a perfect world, but it will continue getting better.

Or perhaps Covid-19 is only a foretaste of even worse to come. Perhaps we'll backslide. If anti-vaccine prophets peddle their deadly disinformation without response, if our last antibiotics are wasted on adding a few ounces of white meat to a chicken breast, if we do nothing to improve global cooperation, surveillance coverage, and rapid response to outbreaks, we know what the world will look like. A planet without our most effective tools against infection is one moving back toward Malthusian misery. It's a world where our view of mortality as an increasingly private affair is blown away by mass burial of the young. It's a world that is poorer, more violent, more insular—a bigoted and misogynistic place.

The role of disease in global affairs has implications for national security: until we reach global targets to reduce nuclear weapons stockpiles close to zero, the most straightforward way for humanity to rapidly roll back decades or even centuries of progress remains the intercontinental ballistic missile. But the world now surely recognizes that pestilence may be the more likely source of a millennial global catastrophe—certainly the First Horseman rides ahead of terror, climate change, or a collapse in food production.

Meanwhile, "neo-Malthusians," concerned with the carrying capacity of the planet, are looking at the wrong threats. For them it is shortage—famine brought on by too many people and not enough resources—that spells doom. But while the threat of global famine may stalk in the rear if we don't move onto a more environmentally sustainable course of production, pestilence remains the more immediate issue. And given that it was lack of technology (rather than of agricultural land) that kept people poor throughout most of history, it makes sense to assume that sustaining the advance of technology is the process by which we'll ensure 9 billion plus people can live on the planet in harmony.

The history of infection teaches a particular lesson to those who want to withdraw from international cooperation: if disease becomes the excuse for closing borders and deploying force, the costs to global progress will be immense. We don't have to accept a new pathogen as the will of God—nor are flight, fortresses, or imprisonment our only defense against the scourge.

Because, for all of the failings and unnecessary deaths of the response to Covid-19, our scientific advances, our health institutions, and global cooperation have put us in an immeasurably better place to fight it than where Petrarch stood with the plague or Montezuma with smallpox. We still face immense risks, but they can be managed without mass coercion. If we use our tools and technologies wisely, there should be little need to resort to the prehistoric defense of exclusion and the dislocation and poverty that accompany it.

Our progress against infection hasn't been an unalloyed good. Not least, it has allowed colonization and total war on a scale unimaginable when imperialists perished in new disease environments and armies wilted under the death rates of typhus and dysentery. But think of a young child—for me, it is one of two daughters. For you it might be a grandchild, cousin, or niece. Now think of that child retching, then vomiting—once, and then again. Imagine her hot to the touch, unable to control her bowels, crying, scared. She becomes weaker, unable to sit up, chest heaving with the struggle of breath. Finally she grows quiet, that silence more fearful than the cries that came before. Her eyes stare listless into space; she's semi-comatose, slipping toward death.

And then think of another child, and imagine it all over again. And then again, five seconds later. And again, twelve times a minute, every minute, of every day. Worldwide, that is about the frequency of under-five deaths. It's a tragedy—and a stain on the world's conscience—that far too many children still die of easily preventable conditions every day. But if we had the global child mortality rate of the 1950s, it would be closer to one death every *second*, five times the level of today—such is the scale of the First Horseman's retreat.

Covid-19 temporarily and tragically reversed progress against infection. But still, far fewer parents than ever before in history go through the pain of burying their own children. The massive decline in premature death is something we should celebrate and protect as humanity's greatest triumph.

Acknowledgments

Many thanks to Rafe Sagalyn for advice and participating in numerous conversations on the shape and structure of the book; Patrick Fitzgerald and Felix Salmon for proposing reorganization and focus; Erle Ellis for insights on land use modeling; Charles C. Mann for detailed and helpful comments and corrections on the early chapters; Paul Offit for reading the text to check for medical mistakes; and Dorothy Porter, Justin Cook, Rodrigo Soares, and David Wootton for catching errors and making suggestions relating to tone and presentation. I apologize for the errors that have slipped under their notice or slipped in since they read drafts. Thanks, too, to Rick Horgan for considerable editorial advice and adjustments.

Notes

Preface

1. Jenny Liu et al., "Malaria Eradication: Is It Possible? Is It Worth It? Should We Do It?" *Lancet Global Health* 1, no. 1 (2013): e2–e3.
2. See David Wootton, *Bad Medicine: Doctors Doing Harm Since Hippocrates* (Oxford, UK: Oxford University Press, 2007); Shapin's review "Possessed by the Idols" in the *London Review of Books* 28, no. 23 (2006), and Wootton's response in the next issue.
3. It's foolish to judge people in the past by modern standards. Ancient doctors didn't all practice malignant quackery and patients clearly saw some value in their services. We can learn much from the "wrong" turns of past scientists—as much as from the "right" ones. Again, that a person invented a medically effective treatment or cure doesn't make them morally pure, and their path to that solution might have involved irrationality or been blazed by means of theories we view today as incorrect. Conversely, people who opposed theories that modern science accepts sometimes did so for reasons that we might find admirable. That said, I don't believe it's an overreach to suggest that lower premature mortality is something that would have been valued in the past or that doctors were frequently seen to be of little use in preventing such mortality. Again, it is not the "judgment of history" that Jenner's development of vaccination was to be celebrated, but the judgment of his contemporaries, including British members of parliament who twice voted him prizes.

Chapter One: Malthus's Ultimate Weapon

1. Thomas Robert Malthus, *An Essay on the Principle of Population; or A View of Its Past and Present Effects on Human Happiness, an Inquiry Into Our Prospects Respecting the Future Removal or Mitigation of the Evils Which It Occasions*, edited with an introduction and notes by Geoffrey Gilbert (Oxford, UK: Oxford University Press, 2008), Chapter VII, p. 61.
2. Recent evidence points to sedentism predating agriculture by as much as three thousand years in the Near East, however, suggesting a complex relationship between the growth of agriculture and cities. Anna Belfer-Cohen and Ofer Bar-Yosef, "Early Sedentism in the Near East," in I. Kuijt (ed.), *Life in Neolithic*

Farming Communities: Fundamental Issues in Archaeology (Boston: Springer, 2002).
3. Max Roser, "Child Mortality," published online at OurWorldInData.org, 2016. Retrieved from https://ourworldindata.org/child-mortality/.
4. Max Roser, "Fertility," published online at OurWorldInData.org, 2016. Retrieved from https://ourworldindata.org/fertility/.
5. Data from the Maddison Project website, http://www.ggdc.net/maddison/maddison-project/home.htm, 2013 version.

Chapter Two: Civilization and the Rise of Infection

1. Analysis also suggests Mitochondrial Eve lived longer ago and some distance from Biblical Eve. In the seventeenth century, Bishop Ussher of the Church of Ireland added up dates and ages in the Old Testament and suggested the world was created on the evening of Sunday, October 22, 4004 BCE. On that basis, Adam's wife came to life only about six thousand years ago. Ewen Callaway, "Genetic Adam and Eve Did Not Live Too Far Apart in Time," *Nature*, August 6, 2013, http://www.nature.com/news/genetic-adam-and-eve-did-not-live-too-far-apart-in-time-1.13478.
2. Mark Nathan Cohen, *Health and the Rise of Civilization* (New Haven: Yale University Press, 1989), p. 18.
3. Rosemary Drisdelle, *Parasites: Tales of Humanity's Most Unwelcome Guests* (Berkeley: University of California Press, 2010).
4. Cohen, *Health and the Rise of Civilization*, pp. 33–35, cross-checked with Nathan D. Wolfe, Claire Panosian Dunavan, and Jared Diamond, "Origins of Major Human Infectious Diseases," *Nature* 447, no. 7142 (2007): 279–283.
5. Cohen, *Health and the Rise of Civilization*, pp. 36–37.
6. See Wolfe et al., "Origins of Major Human Infectious Diseases."
7. Modern Stone Age populations have infant mortality rates largely below (and often considerably below) 25 percent—far lower than rates across Europe and the Americas for much of the nineteenth century. And these rates are likely higher than prehistoric rates because modern hunter-gatherer groups have been subject to most of the diseases of civilization. Cohen, *Health and the Rise of Civilization*, pp. 82–84, 100–101.
8. Cohen, *Health and the Rise of Civilization*, pp. 195–197.
9. Renee Pennington, "Hunter-Gatherer Demography," in Panter-Brick et al., *Hunter-Gatherers: An Interdisciplinary Perspective* (Cambridge, UK: Cambridge University Press, 2001), p. 170.
10. Cohen, *Health and the Rise of Civilization* , pp. 87–88.
11. Azar Gat, "Proving Communal Warfare Among Hunter-Gatherers: The Quasi-Rousseauan Error," *Evolutionary Anthropology: Issues, News, and Reviews* 24, no. 3 (2015): 111–126.
12. See Siniša Malešević, "How Old Is Human Brutality? On the Structural Origins of Violence," *Common Knowledge* 22, no. 1 (2016): 81–104, for a discussion.
13. Vanina Guernier, Michael E. Hochberg, and Jean-François Guégan, "Ecology

Drives the Worldwide Distribution of Human Diseases," *PLoS Biol* 2, no. 6 (2004): e141.

14. Robert R. Dunn et al., "Global Drivers of Human Pathogen Richness and Prevalence," *Proceedings of the Royal Society of London B: Biological Sciences* (April 2010).
15. William McNeill, *Plagues and Peoples* (New York: Anchor, 1996). Certainly, Native Americans on the plains of North America in the nineteenth century were among the tallest people in the world—the health that suggests reflecting not least the low natural disease burden of a sparsely populated hunting ground. Richard H. Steckel and Joseph M. Prince, "Tallest in the World: Native Americans of the Great Plains in the Nineteenth Century," *American Economic Review* 91, no. 1 (March 2001): 287.
16. McNeill, *Plagues and Peoples.*
17. Herbert S. Klein, "The First Americans: The Current Debate," *Journal of Interdisciplinary History* 46, no. 4 (2016): 543–562. The theory is disputed (see L. Nagaoka, T. Rick, and S. Wolverton, "The Overkill Model and Its Impact on Environmental Research," *Ecology and Evolution* 8, no. 19 [2018]: 9683–9696), and there was also a role for climate change (see Anthony D. Barnosky and Emily L. Lindsey, "Timing of Quaternary Megafaunal Extinction in South America in Relation to Human Arrival and Climate Change," *Quaternary International* 217, nos. 1–2 [2010]: 10–29).
18. See Exodus 9:14–15.
19. James C. Scott, *Against the Grain: A Deep History of the First Civilizations* (New Haven: Yale University Press, 2017).
20. There is still some debate as to whether malaria infected pre-civilization humans. Certainly not all strains did, but some may have—see the discussion in Dorothy Crawford, *Deadly Companions: How Microbes Shaped Our History* (Oxford, UK: Oxford University Press, 2007), pp. 37–46, and Monica Green, "The Globalisations of Disease," in N. Boivin, R. Crassard, and M. Petraglia (eds.), *Human Dispersal and Species Movement: From Prehistory to the Present* (Cambridge, UK: Cambridge University Press, 2017), pp. 494–520.
21. Crawford, *Deadly Companions*, p. 68.
22. Ibid., p. 60.
23. IRIN News, "Pig-Cull Induced Street Rubbish 'National Scandal,'" January 26, 2010. Retrieved from http://www.irinnews.org/report/87853/egypt-pig-cull-induced-street-rubbish-a-national-scandal.
24. Drisdelle, *Parasites.*
25. Ibid.
26. Kelly Harkins and Anne Stone, "Ancient Pathogen Genomics: Insights into Timing and Adaptation," *Journal of Human Evolution* 79 (2015): 137–49.
27. Wolfe et al., "Origins of Major Human Infectious Diseases," and Harkins and Stone, "Ancient Pathogen Genomics."
28. J. O. Wertheim, M. D. Smith, D. M. Smith, K. Scheffler, and S. L. Kosakovsky Pond, "Evolutionary Origins of Human Herpes Simplex Viruses 1 and 2," *Molecular Biology and Evolution* 31, no. 9 (2014): 2356–2364. Hepatitis B and an early form of tuberculosis are other examples. Andrew P. Dobson and E. Robin

Carper, "Infectious Diseases and Human Population History," *Bioscience* 46, no. 2 (1996): 115–126, Green, "Globalisations of Disease."

29. Scott, *Against the Grain*, p. 4.
30. Yuki Furuse, Akira Suzuki, and Hitoshi Oshitani, "Origin of Measles Virus: Divergence from Rinderpest Virus between the 11th and 12th Centuries," *Virology Journal* 7, no. 52 (2010).
31. Dobson and Carper, "Infectious Diseases."
32. Furuse, "Origin of Measles Virus."
33. Sarah Cobey, "Modeling Infectious Disease Dynamics," *Science*, April 24, 2020.
34. Marcus J. Hamilton, Robert S. Walker, and Dylan C. Kesler, "Crash and Rebound of Indigenous Populations in Lowland South America," *Scientific Reports* 4 (2014).
35. Deepa Naraya et al., *Voices of the Poor: Can Anyone Hear Us?* (New York: Oxford University Press, 2000).
36. Peter Katona and Judit Katona-Apte, "The Interaction Between Nutrition and Infection," *Clinical Infectious Diseases* 46, no. 10 (2008): 1582–1588. For a summary of the debate over the related McKeown Thesis, see James Colgrove, "The McKeown Thesis: A Historical Controversy and Its Enduring Influence," *American Journal of Public Health* 92, no. 5 (2002): 725–729.
37. Cohen, *Health and the Rise of Civilization*, pp. 58–64.
38. Ibid., pp. 116–124. See also Richard H. Steckel, *The Best of Times, the Worst of Times: Health and Nutrition in Pre-Columbian America*, Working Paper no.10299, National Bureau of Economic Research, 2004.
39. Simon Szreter, "The Importance of Social Intervention in Britain's Mortality Decline c. 1850–1914: A Re-interpretation of the Role of Public Health," *Social History of Medicine* 1, no. 1 (1988): 1–38, on Liverpool. Data on life expectancy from Gapminder for Sierra Leone is 25.1 and Nigeria 30.4 for 1850, for example (from www.gapminder.org).
40. In addition, the average height of recruits to the British Army fell between the 1820s and the 1850s, led by city recruits. Bernard Harris, "Public Health, Nutrition, and the Decline of Mortality: The McKeown Thesis Revisited," *Social History of Medicine* 17, no. 3 (2004): 379–407.
41. As the Biblical God had warned Biblical Eve on her exile from Eden: "I will greatly multiply thy sorrow and thy conception; in sorrow thou shalt bring forth children; and thy desire shall be to thy husband, and he shall rule over thee" (Genesis 3:16).
42. Note the order between fertility leading to population growth leading to infection (as opposed to population growth from other causes leading to infection creating pressure to increase fertility) is debatable. See Jean-Pierre Bocquet-Appel, "When the World's Population Took Off: The Springboard of the Neolithic Demographic Transition," *Science* 333, no. 6042 (2011): 560–561.
43. Scott, *Against the Grain*, p. 82, suggests it is not just "domesticated" humans who experience higher fertility—the same occurs with rats and foxes.
44. *The Code of Hammurabi*, translated by L. W. King. Retrieved from http://avalon.law.yale.edu/ancient/hamframe.asp.
45. Ester Boserup, *The Conditions of Agricultural Growth: The Economics of Agrarian Change Under Population Pressure* (London: George Allen and Unwin, 1965), p. 4.

46. Ibid., p. 7.
47. Ibid., p. 30.
48. See Jed Kaplan et al., "Holocene Carbon Emissions as a Result of Anthropogenic Land Cover Change," *Holocene* 1 (2010): 17, and Kees Klein Goldewijk et al., "The HYDE 3.1 Spatially Explicit Database of Human-Induced Global Land-Use Change over the Past 12,000 Years," *Global Ecology and Biogeography* 20, no.1 (2011): 73–86.
49. Cormac Ó Gráda, *Famine: A Short History* (Princeton, NJ: Princeton University Press, 2009).
50. Walter Scheidel, "Emperors, Aristocrats, and the Grim Reaper: Towards a Demographic Profile of the Roman Elite," *Classical Quarterly* 49, no. 1 (1999): 254–281.
51. Scott, *Against the Grain*, p. 35.
52. Data available from the Yale University SETO lab: http://urban.yale.edu/data.

Chapter Three: Trade Merges Disease Pools

1. James C. Scott, *Against the Grain: A Deep History of the First Civilizations* (New Haven: Yale University Press, 2017), p. 125.
2. Mark Nathan Cohen, *Health and the Rise of Civilization* (New Haven: Yale University Press, 1989), p. 23.
3. William Bernstein, *A Splendid Exchange: How Trade Shaped the World* (New York: Grove/Atlantic, Inc., 2009), pp. 44–45 and 49.
4. M. J. Papagrigorakis et al., "DNA Examination of Ancient Dental Pulp Incriminates Typhoid Fever as a Probable Cause of the Plague of Athens," *International Journal of Infectious Diseases* 10, no. 3 (2006): 206–214, and Powel Kazanjian, "Ebola in Antiquity?" *Clinical Infectious Diseases* 61, no. 6 (September 2015): 963–968.
5. Thucydides, *The History of the Peloponnesian War*, translated by Richard Crawley, Chapter VII. Retrieved from http://classics.mit.edu/Thucydides/pelopwar.2.second.html.
6. Arnold Toynbee, *A Study of History*, abridgement of Vols. I–VI by D. C. Somervell (Cambridge, UK: Oxford University Press, 1974), pp. 183–184.
7. Livy's *History of Rome: Book 3*, translated by Rev. Canon Roberts. Retrieved from http://mcadams.posc.mu.edu/txt/ah/Livy/Livy03.html.
8. Frederick Fox Cartwright and Michael Denis Biddiss, *Disease and History* (New York: Marboro Books, 1972), p. 10.
9. Scott, *Against the Grain*, p. 156.
10. Quoted in Raoul McLaughlin, *Rome and the Distant East: Trade Routes to the Ancient Lands of Arabia, India and China* (London: Bloomsbury Publishing, 2010), p. 3.
11. McNeill, *Plagues and Peoples*.
12. William Rosen, *Justinian's Flea: Plague, Empire and the Birth of Europe* (New York: Random House, 2010).
13. Yu Huan, *The Peoples of the West* from the *Weilue*, a third-century Chinese account composed between 239 and 265 CE, quoted in *zhuan* 30 of the *Sanguozhi*,

published in 429 CE, English translation by John E. Hill. Retrieved from http://depts.washington.edu/silkroad/texts/weilue/weilue.html.

14. Kyle Harper, *The Fate of Rome: Climate, Disease, and the End of an Empire* (Princeton, NJ: Princeton University Press, 2017).
15. Cartwright and Biddiss, *Disease and History*, p. 13.
16. R. S. Bray, *Armies of Pestilence: The Impact of Disease on History* (Cambridge, UK: James Clarke & Co., 2004), pp. 12–13.
17. Kyle Harper, "Pandemics and Passages to Late Antiquity: Rethinking the Plague of c. 249–270 Described by Cyprian," *Journal of Roman Archaeology* 28 (2015): 223–260.
18. Robert Sallares, Abigail Bouwman, and Cecilia Anderung, "The Spread of Malaria to Southern Europe in Antiquity: New Approaches to Old Problems," *Medical History* 48, no. 3 (2004): 311–328.
19. Procopius of Caesarea, "The Secret History," translated by Richard Atwater. Fordham University Medieval Sourcebook. Retrieved from http://www.fordham.edu/halsall/source/procop-anec1.asp.
20. Ibid.
21. Nicolás Rascovan, Karl-Göran Sjögren, Kristian Kristiansen, Rasmus Nielsen, Eske Willerslev, Christelle Desnues, and Simon Rasmussen, "Emergence and Spread of Basal Lineages of Yersinia Pestis During the Neolithic Decline," *Cell* 176, nos. 1–2 (2019): 295–305.
22. Bernstein, *A Splendid Exchange*, p. 139.
23. Monica Green, "Taking 'Pandemic' Seriously: Making the Black Death Global," *Medieval Globe* 1, no. 1 (2016).
24. M. Harbeck et al., "*Yersinia pestis* DNA from Skeletal Remains from the 6th Century CE Reveals Insights into Justinianic Plague," *PLoS Pathogens* 9, no. 5 (2013).
25. Quoted in Lester K. Little, "Life and Afterlife of the First Plague Pandemic," in Lester K. Little (ed.), *Plague and the End of Antiquity* (Cambridge, UK: Cambridge University Press, 2007), p. 7.
26. Procopius, *History of the Wars*, Books I and II. Retrieved from http://www.gutenberg.org/files/16764/16764-h/16764-h.htm.
27. Bray, *Armies of Pestilence*, p. 42.
28. Procopius of Caesarea, "The Secret History."
29. Bray, *Armies of Pestilence*, p. 29, and Rosen, *Justinian's Flea*.
30. Bray, *Armies of Pestilence*, p. 116.
31. Bernstein, *A Splendid Exchange*, p. 137.
32. John Kelly, *The Great Mortality: An Intimate History of the Black Death, the Most Devastating Plague of All Time* (New York: HarperCollins, 2005), p. 44.
33. Little, "Life and Afterlife," and Rosen, *Justinian's Flea*.
34. Forest cover in England and Germany may have fallen to below 10 percent in 1350. Jed O. Kaplan, Kristen M. Krumhardt, and Niklaus Zimmermann, "The Prehistoric and Preindustrial Deforestation of Europe," *Quaternary Science Reviews* 28, no. 27 (2009): 3016–3034.
35. Kelly, *The Great Mortality*.
36. Quoted by Ronald Latham in his Introduction to *Marco Polo: The Travels* (New York: Penguin, 1958), p. 11.

37. Marco Polo, *The Travels*, translated by Ronald Latham, pp. 57, 66, and 80.
38. Quoted in Roger Crowley, *City of Fortune: How Venice Ruled the Seas* (New York: Random House, 2012).
39. Polo, *The Travels*, pp. 150–151.
40. Ibid., p. 98.
41. Quoted in Mark Wheelis, "Biological Warfare at the 1346 Siege of Caffa," *Emerging Infectious Diseases* 8, no. 9 (2002): 971–975.
42. Kelly, *The Great Mortality*, and Wheelis, "Biological Warfare," provide reasons for some skepticism on the role of Caffa refugees in spreading the plague onward.
43. From Boccaccio, *The Decameron*, translated by J. M. Rigg, 1903. Available at https://www.brown.edu/Departments/Italian_Studies/dweb/texts/.
44. "Letters on Familiar Matters," in John Aberth, *The Black Death: The Great Mortality of 1348–1350: A Brief History with Documents* (London: Palgrave Macmillan, 2005).
45. Quoted in Kelly, *The Great Mortality*, p. 145.
46. José Gómez and Miguel Verdú, "Network Theory May Explain the Vulnerability of Medieval Human Settlements to the Black Death Pandemic," *Nature Scientific Reports* 7 (2017): 43467.
47. Petrarch, *Petrarca Ad Seipsum*, Volume I, Chapter 14, translated by Jonathan Usher, University of Edinburgh. Retrieved from http://www.brown.edu/Departments/Italian_Studies/dweb/plague/perspectives/petrarca2.php.
48. Quoted in Aberth, "Letters on Familiar Matters," p. 72.
49. Sheldon Watts, *Epidemics and History: Disease, Power and Imperialism* (New Haven: Yale University Press, 1999), p. 3.
50. Kelly, *The Great Mortality*, p. 248.
51. Cartwright and Biddis, *Disease and History*, p. 47.
52. Bray, *Armies of Pestilence*, p. 69.
53. Jo Nelson Hays, *The Burdens of Disease: Epidemics and Human Response in Western History* (New Brunswick, NJ: Rutgers University Press, 2009), p. 46.
54. UK Government, "Ordinance of Laborers," 1349, Fordham University Sourcebook. Retrieved from http://legacy.fordham.edu/halsall/seth/ordinance-labourers.asp.
55. Kelly, *The Great Mortality*.
56. Norman F. Cantor, *In the Wake of the Plague: The Black Death and the World It Made* (New York: Simon & Schuster, 2001).
57. Additionally, wages for women's casual employment did increase after the plague, which might have been an incentive for married women to substitute child-rearing for working. Jane Humphries and Jacob Weisdorf, "The Wages of Women in England, 1260–1850," *Journal of Economic History* 75, no. 2 (June 2015): 405–447.
58. Margaret Peters, "Labor Markets After the Black Death: Landlord Collusion and the Imposition of Serfdom in Eastern Europe and the Middle East," mimeo, prepared for the Stanford Comparative Politics Workshop, 2010.
59. Gregory Clark, *A Farewell to Alms: A Brief Economic History of the World* (Princeton, NJ: Princeton University Press, 2007), estimates that income per person in the UK more than doubled between the 1310s and the 1450s.
60. G. D. Sussman, "Was the Black Death in India and China?" *Bulletin of the History of Medicine*, 2011, pp. 319–355.

61. Giovanna Morelli, Yajun Song, Camila J. Mazzoni, Mark Eppinger, Philippe Roumagnac, David M. Wagner, Mirjam Feldkamp et al., "Yersinia Pestis Genome Sequencing Identifies Patterns of Global Phylogenetic Diversity," *Nature Genetics* 42, no. 12 (2010): 1140–1143.
62. Christian E. Demeure, Olivier Dussurget, Guillem Mas Fiol, Anne-Sophie Le Guern, Cyril Savin, and Javier Pizarro-Cerdá, "Yersinia Pestis and Plague: An Updated View on Evolution, Virulence Determinants, Immune Subversion, Vaccination, and Diagnostics," *Genes & Immunity* 20, no. 5 (2019): 357–370.
63. Nico Voigtländer and Hans-Joachim Voth, "The Three Horsemen of Riches: Plague, War, and Urbanization in Early Modern Europe," *Review of Economic Studies* 80, no. 2 (2012): 774–811.
64. Cartwright and Biddis, *Disease and History*, p. 32.

Chapter Four: Pestilence Conquers

1. Bastien Llamas, Lars Fehren-Schmitz, Guido Valverde, Julien Soubrier, Swapan Mallick, Nadin Rohland, Susanne Nordenfelt et al., "Ancient Mitochondrial DNA Provides High-Resolution Time Scale of the Peopling of the Americas," *Science Advances* 2, no. 4 (2016).
2. Anthony D. Barnosky and Emily L. Lindsey, "Timing of Quaternary Megafaunal Extinction in South America in Relation to Human Arrival and Climate Change," *Quaternary International* 217, nos. 1–2 (2010): 10–29, discuss the roles of climate and human activities; Zachary D. Nickell and Matthew D. Moran, "Disease Introduction by Aboriginal Humans in North America and the Pleistocene Extinction," *Journal of Ecological Anthropology* 19, no. 1 (2017): 2, the role of introduced disease.
3. Dorothy Crawford, *Deadly Companions: How Microbes Shaped Our History* (Oxford, UK: Oxford University Press, 2007), pp. 112–113. The reason for the caveat of "mostly" is recent evidence suggesting that at least human tuberculosis was present before Columbus, potentially brought to the Americas via seals (Kirsten I. Bos et al., "Pre-Columbian Mycobacterial Genomes Reveal Seals as a Source of New World Human Tuberculosis," *Nature* 514 [2014]: 494).
4. W. M. Denevan, "After 1492: Nature Rebounds," *Geographical Review* 106, no. 3 (2016): 381–398, and Angus Maddison, *The World Economy, Volume 1: A Millennial Perspective* and *Volume 2: Historical Statistics* (Haryana, India: Academic Foundation, 2007).
5. Charles C. Mann, *1491: New Revelations of the Americas Before Columbus* (New York: Alfred A. Knopf, 2005).
6. Ibid., p. 72.
7. Ibid., p. 140.
8. Latham, introduction to *Marco Polo: The Travels*.
9. William Bernstein, *A Splendid Exchange: How Trade Shaped the World* (New York: Grove/Atlantic, Inc., 2009), p. 166.
10. Christopher Columbus, *The Four Voyages of Christopher Columbus*, translated by John Cohen (London: Penguin UK, 1969), pp. 58–59.
11. Ibid., p. 122.

12. Noble David Cook, *Born to Die: Disease and New World Conquest, 1492–1650* (Cambridge, UK: Cambridge University Press, 1998), pp. 57–58.
13. R. S. Bray, *Armies of Pestilence: The Impact of Disease on History* (Cambridge, UK: James Clarke & Co., 2004), pp. 125, and Mark Harrison, *Disease and the Modern World: 1500 to the Present Day* (New York: John Wiley & Sons, 2013), p. 73.
14. Sheldon Watts, *Epidemics and History: Disease, Power and Imperialism* (New Haven: Yale University Press, 1999), p. 89.
15. Quoted in Hugh Thomas, *Conquest: Cortés, Montezuma, and the Fall of Old Mexico* (New York: Simon & Schuster, 2013).
16. Quoted in Watts, *Epidemics and History*, p. 89.
17. Las Casas, *A Short Account of the Destruction of the Indes*. Retrieved from http://nationalhumanitiescenter.org/pds/amerbegin/contact/text7/casas_destruction.pdf.
18. Mann, *1491: New Revelations of the Americas*, p. 61.
19. Ibid.
20. Ibid.
21. Watts, *Epidemics and History*, p. 93.
22. Ibid., p. 233.
23. Quoted in ibid., p. 235.
24. See Philip D. Curtin, *Death by Migration: Europe's Encounter with the Tropical World in the Nineteenth Century* (Cambridge, UK: Cambridge University Press, 1989), for a discussion.
25. Elena Esposito, *Side Effects of Immunities: The African Slave Trade*, Working Paper no. MWP2015/09, European University Institute, 2015.
26. Robert A. McGuire and Philip Coelho, *Parasites, Pathogens, and Progress* (Cambridge, MA: MIT Press, 2011), Chapter 5.
27. Bray, *Armies of Pestilence*, p. 129.
28. Malthus's estimate was from Benjamin Franklin, who wrote an article on demographics in the 1750s. Personal communication from Charles Mann.
29. His ignorance of the role of disease in creating the wide open spaces of the Americas is clear from his discussion of Central America. (Thomas Robert Malthus, *An Essay on the Principle of Population; or a View of Its Past and Present Effects on Human Happiness, an Inquiry Into Our Prospects Respecting the Future Removal Or Mitigation of the Evils which it Occasions*, edited with an introduction and notes by Geoffrey Gilbert [Oxford, UK: Oxford University Press, 2008], Chapter VI, paragraph I.)
30. Louis Putterman, and David N. Weil, *Post-1500 Population Flows and the Long Run Determinants of Economic Growth and Inequality*, no. w14448, National Bureau of Economic Research, 2008.
31. King Afonso I, letter to King John III of Portugal, 1526. Retrieved from https://mrcaseyhistory.files.wordpress.com/2014/05/king-afonso-i-letter-to-king-john-iii-of-portugal.pdf.
32. Population estimates from the Maddison Project website, http://www.ggdc.net/maddison/oriindex.htm.
33. Philip Curtin et al., *African History from Earliest Times to Independence* (New York: Pearson, 1995).
34. Stanley L. Engerman and Kenneth L. Sokoloff, in *Factor Endowments, Inequality, and Paths of Development Among New World Economics*, no. w9259, National Bu-

reau of Economic Research, 2002, argue that it wasn't so much the risk of death to colonists that shaped the population makeup of colonies, it was more the nature of the land they colonized. In the tropics, colonies were built on a model of exploiting slaves or natives in mines or on large plantations growing crops like sugar and tobacco. Outside the tropics, the crops that did well could be grown on small farms as successfully as they could on large ones, so demand for slave labor was lower and homesteading made sense. As the areas where tropical diseases were the greatest threat and the areas where plantation farming made sense largely overlap, the stories reinforce each other.

35. Nathan Nunn, "The Long-Term Effects of Africa's Slave Trades," *Quarterly Journal of Economics* 1, no. 23 (2008): 139–176, and Nathan Nunn and Leonard Wantchekon, "The Slave Trade and the Origins of Mistrust in Africa," *American Economic Review* 101 (2011): 3221–3252.
36. Stelios Michalopoulos and Elias Papaioannou, "Further Evidence on the Link Between Pre-Colonial Political Centralization and Comparative Economic Development in Africa," *Economics Letters* 126 (2015): 57–62.
37. Patrick Manson, "The Malaria Parasite," *Journal of the Royal African Society* 6, no. 23 (1907): 225–233.
38. There is argument over the New World status of the disease (see for example Watts, *Epidemics and History* p. 130), but some evidence suggests both that it was present in the Americas before Columbus's arrival (see Bruce M. Rothschild et al., "First European Exposure to Syphilis: The Dominican Republic at the Time of Columbian Contact," *Clinical Infectious Diseases* 31, no. 4 [2000]: 936–941) and that the disease is most closely related to a variation of yaws found in Guyana (Kristin N. Harper et al., "On the Origin of the Treponematoses: A Phylogenetic Approach," *PLoS Neglected Tropical Diseases* 2, no. 1 [2008]).
39. Hans Zinsser, *Rats, Lice and History* (Piscataway, NJ: Transaction Publishers, 2007), p. 75.
40. Jo Nelson Hays, *The Burdens of Disease: Epidemics and Human Response in Western History* (New Brunswick, NJ: Rutgers University Press, 2009), p. 70, and Dorothy Crawford, *Deadly Companions: How Microbes Shaped Our History* (Oxford, UK: Oxford University Press, 2007), p. 125.
41. Frederick Fox Cartwright and Michael Denis Biddiss, *Disease and History* (New York: Marboro Books, 1972), p. 63.
42. A. B. Jannetta, *Epidemics and Mortality in Early Modern Japan* (Princeton, NJ: Princeton University Press, 2014).
43. A. Jannetta, "Jennerian Vaccination and the Creation of a National Public Health Agenda in Japan, 1850–1900," *Bulletin of the History of Medicine* 83, no. 1 (2009): 125–140.
44. Zinsser *Rats, Lice and History*, p. 152.
45. Ibid., pp. 155–156.
46. Ibid., p. 168.
47. Bray, *Armies of Pestilence*, p. 139.
48. Harrison, *Disease and the Modern World*, p. 84.
49. Michael B. A. Oldstone, *Viruses, Plagues, and History: Past, Present, and Future* (Oxford, UK: Oxford University Press. 2009), p. 107.

50. Joseph M. Conlon, *The Historical Impact of Epidemic Typhus*. Retrieved from http://phthiraptera.info/sites/phthiraptera.info/files/61235.pdf.
51. Jakob Walter, *Diary of a Napoleonic Foot Soldier* (New York: Doubleday, 2012), p. 43.
52. Stephan Talty, *The Illustrious Dead: The Terrifying Story of How Typhus Killed Napoleon's Greatest Army* (New York: Crown Publishers, 2009), p. 62.
53. Talty, *The Illustrious Dead*, p. 84.
54. Ibid., p. 156.
55. Walter, *Diary of a Napoleonic Foot Soldier*, p. 57.
56. Ibid., pp. 62–63.
57. Ibid., p. 78.
58. Didier Raoult et al., "Evidence for Louse-Transmitted Diseases in Soldiers of Napoleon's Grand Army in Vilnius," *Journal of Infectious Diseases* 193, no. 1 (2006): 112–120.
59. Bray, *Armies of Pestilence*, p. 146.

Chapter Five: The Exclusion Instinct

1. See the enjoyable discussion in Matt Ridley, *The Red Queen: Sex and the Evolution of Human Nature* (London: Penguin UK, 1994).
2. It seems hard to explain (for example) the hideous death toll that Polynesians first exposed to measles suffered in the nineteenth century—approaching 80 percent—without factoring in a lower level of genetic resistance. Robert A. McGuire and Philip Coelho, *Parasites, Pathogens, and Progress* (Cambridge, MA: MIT Press, 2011). See also Elinor K. Karlsson, Dominic P. Kwiatkowski, and Pardis C. Sabeti, "Natural Selection and Infectious Disease in Human Populations," *Nature Reviews Genetics* 15, no. 6 (2014): 379.
3. Andrew Spielman and Michael d'Antonio, *Mosquito: The Story of Man's Deadliest Foe* (New York: Hyperion, 2002).
4. Frédéric B. Piel et al., "Global Distribution of the Sickle Cell Gene and Geographical Confirmation of the Malaria Hypothesis," *Nature Communications* 1 (2010): 104.
5. See Karlsson et al., "Natural Selection and Infectious Disease." R. S. Bray, *Armies of Pestilence: The Impact of Disease on History* (Cambridge, UK: James Clarke & Co., 2004), p. 37, notes another potential channel for resistance to infection, through the immunoglobulin G, an antibody that can pass temporary immunity from mother to child across the placenta. If the child is infected before he or she has destroyed the inherited immunoglobulin, it will help the child survive the disease and develop longer-term resistance.
6. Valerie Curtis et al., "Disgust as an Adaptive System for Disease Avoidance Behavior," *Philosophical Transactions of the Royal Society of London. Series B, Biological Sciences* 366, no. 1563 (2011): 389–401.
7. Quoted in Hans Zinsser, *Rats, Lice and History* (Piscataway, NJ: Transaction Publishers, 2007), p. 138.
8. Benjamin L. Hart, "Behavioral Adaptations to Pathogens and Parasites: Five Strategies," *Neuroscience & Biobehavioral Reviews* 14, no. 3 (1990): 273–294.

9. Sarah Cobey, "Modeling Infectious Disease Dynamics," *Science*, April 24, 2020.
10. Kyla Epstein, "Just 14% of Americans Support Ending Social Distancing," *Business Insider*, April 22, 2020, https://www.businessinsider.com/poll-most-americans-support-coronavirus-social-distancing-measures-2020-4, and Alexis Le Nestour, "Five Findings from a New Phone Survey in Senegal," Center for Global Development blog, April 24, 2020, https://www.cgdev.org/blog/five-findings-new-phone-survey-senegal.
11. Chad R. Mortensen et al., "Infection Breeds Reticence: The Effects of Disease Salience on Self-Perceptions of Personality and Behavioral Avoidance Tendencies," *Psychological Science* 21 (2010): 440–447.
12. Alan M. Kraut, "Foreign Bodies: The Perennial Negotiation over Health and Culture in a Nation of Immigrants," *Journal of American Ethnic History* (2004): 3–22.
13. James C. Scott, *Against the Grain: A Deep History of the First Civilizations* (New Haven: Yale University Press, 2017), p. 99.
14. Jeanette Farrell, *Invisible Enemies: Stories of Infectious Disease* (New York: Farrar Straus and Giroux, 1998), p. 62.
15. Leprosy Mission, "Diana Princess of Wales," published online at the Leprosy Mission website, http://www.leprosymission.org.uk/about-us-and-leprosy/our-history/diana-princess-of-wales.aspx.
16. Liang Huigang, Xiang Xiaowei, Huang Cui, Ma Haixia, and Yuan Zhiming, "A Brief History of the Development of Infectious Disease Prevention, Control, and Biosafety Programs in China," *Journal of Biosafety and Biosecurity* 2, no. 2 (2020).
17. Dorothy Porter, *Health, Civilization and the State: A History of Public Health from Ancient to Modern Times* (Abingdon, UK: Routledge, 2005), p. 29.
18. Sheldon Watts, *Epidemics and History: Disease, Power and Imperialism* (New Haven: Yale University Press, 1999), p. 50, and Porter, *Health, Civilization and the State*, p. 29.
19. Watts, *Epidemics and History*, p. 52.
20. Ibid., p. 49. In addition, perhaps legitimate cases of the condition became less common in the years after the plague. The spread of tuberculosis may have rendered the one in ten (approximately) who are ever susceptible to Hansen's disease immune. Porter, *Health, Civilization and the State*, p. 28.
21. Nico Voigtländer and Hans-Joachim Voth, "The Three Horsemen of Riches: Plague, War, and Urbanization in Early Modern Europe," *Review of Economic Studies* 80, no. 2 (2012): 774–811.
22. Ibid.
23. Jo Nelson Hays, *The Burdens of Disease: Epidemics and Human Response in Western History* (New Brunswick, NJ: Rutgers University Press, 2009), pp. 54–55, and Watts, *Epidemics and History*, p. 22.
24. Porter, *Health, Civilization and the State*, p. 37.
25. Eugenia Tognotti, "Lessons from the History of Quarantine, from Plague to Influenza A," *Emerging Infectious Diseases* 19, no. 2 (2013): 254.
26. From Boccaccio, *The Decameron*, translated by J. M. Rigg (1903). Available at https://www.brown.edu/Departments/Italian_Studies/dweb/texts/.
27. Mark Nathan Cohen, *Health and the Rise of Civilization* (New Haven: Yale University Press, 1989), p. 53.

28. Mark Harrison, *Disease and the Modern World: 1500 to the Present Day* (New York: John Wiley & Sons, 2013), p. 44.
29. John Kelly, *The Great Mortality: An Intimate History of the Black Death, the Most Devastating Plague of All Time* (New York: HarperCollins, 2005), Chapter 5.
30. Porter, *Health, Civilization and the State*, pp. 34–35.
31. Watts, *Epidemics and History*, p. 24.
32. David M. Morens, Gregory K. Folkers, and Anthony S. Fauci, "Emerging Infections: A Perpetual Challenge," *Lancet Infectious Diseases* 8, no. 11 (2008): 710–719.
33. Watts, *Epidemics and History*, p. 137.
34. Fahd Khan et al., "The Story of the Condom," *Indian Journal of Urology: Journal of the Urological Society of India* 29, no. 1 (2013): 12.
35. Ibid.
36. Edward H. Beardsley, "Allied Against Sin: American and British Responses to Venereal Disease in World War I," *Medical History* 20, no. 2 (1976): 189–202.
37. Cited in Farrell, *Invisible Enemies*, pp. 183–184.
38. Porter, *Health, Civilization and the State*, p. 135.
39. Hays, *The Burdens of Disease*, p. 172.
40. Porter, *Health, Civilization and the State*, p. 137.
41. Howard Markel and Alexandra Minna Stern, "The Foreignness of Germs: The Persistent Association of Immigrants and Disease in American Society," *Milbank Quarterly* 80, no. 4 (2002): 757–788.
42. Hays, *The Burdens of Disease*, p. 185.
43. Kraut, *Foreign Bodies*.
44. Hays, *The Burdens of Disease*, p. 303.
45. Markel and Stern, "The Foreignness of Germs."
46. Adam Nossiter, "Fear of Ebola Breeds a Terror of Physicians," *New York Times*, July 27, 2014. Retrieved from http://www.nytimes.com/2014/07/28/world/africa/ebola-epidemic-west-africa-guinea.html.
47. Amy Brittan, "The Women Chanted to the Village's Men . . . ," *Washington Post*, January 1, 2015, p. 1.
48. Jamelle Bouie, "America's Long History of Immigrant Scaremongering," *Slate*, July 18, 2014, http://www.slate.com/articles/news_and_politics/politics/2014/07/immigrant_scaremongering_and_hate_conservatives_stoke_fears_of_diseased.html.
49. Ibid.
50. Mark Schaller and Damian Murray, "Infectious Disease and the Creation of Culture," *Advances in Culture and Psychology* 1 (2011): 99–151. See also Florian van Leeuwen et al., "Regional Variation in Pathogen Prevalence Predicts Endorsement of Group-Focused Moral Concerns," *Evolution and Human Behavior* 33 (2012). Although note Elizabeth Cashdan and Matthew Steele, "Pathogen Prevalence, Group Bias, and Collectivism in the Standard Cross-Cultural Sample," *Human Nature* 24, no. 1 (2013): 59–75.
51. Cullen S. Hendrix and Kristian Skrede Gleditsch, "Civil War: Is It All About Disease and Xenophobia? A Comment on Letendre, Fincher & Thornhill," *Biological Reviews* 87, no. 1 (2012): 163–167.

52. So far, the researchers working on parasite stress haven't been able to convincingly demonstrate that it is the behavioral response to communicable disease that dominates in the relationship between quality of life and levels of infection. The best they have managed is to note that measures of parasite stress dating back to the 1930s are related to current levels of violence, xenophobia, and so on. But countries that were healthier, richer, and more peaceful in the 1930s remain healthier, richer, and more peaceful today, so that the relationship holds between modern development outcomes and seventy-year-old parasite stress isn't fully reassuring as evidence of what causes what. Even if parasites play a role in violence and distrust, it might be through more the direct impact of illness or some other mechanism than greater distrust of strangers. For example, Matteo Cervellati et al., *Malaria Risk and Civil Violence*, Munich Discussion Paper 2017–8, University of Munich, suggest that malaria outbreaks are linked to civil unrest because they cause sizeable economic losses through incapacity and medical payments rather than through any change in attitudes.

Chapter Six: Cleaning Up

1. Paul W. Sherman and Jennifer Billing, "Darwinian Gastronomy: Why We Use Spices," *BioScience* 49, no. 6 (1999): 453–463.
2. Mark Schaller and Damian Murray, "Infectious Disease and the Creation of Culture," *Advances in Culture and Psychology* 1 (2011).
3. W. Hodding Carter, *Flushed: How the Plumber Saved Civilization* (New York: Simon & Schuster, 2006), pp. 25–26.
4. Marco Polo, *The Travels*, translated by Ronald Latham (New York: Penguin, 1958), pp. 213–222.
5. Ibid., pp. 130 and 136.
6. Lord Amulree, "Hygienic Conditions in Ancient Rome and Modern London," *Medical History* 17.3 (1973): 244–255.
7. Frederick Fox Cartwright and Michael Denis Biddiss, *Disease and History* (New York: Marboro Books, 1972), p. 23.
8. St. Jerome, *Letters*, No. 107: To Laeta. Retrieved from New Advent, http://www.newadvent.org/fathers/3001107.htm.
9. John Kelly, *The Great Mortality: An Intimate History of the Black Death, the Most Devastating Plague of All Time* (New York: HarperCollins, 2005).
10. Nico Voigtländer and Hans-Joachim Voth, "The Three Horsemen of Riches: Plague, War, and Urbanization in Early Modern Europe," *Review of Economic Studies* 80, no. 2 (2013): 774–811.
11. Quoted in D. Evans, "A Good Riddance of Bad Rubbish? Scatological Musings on Rubbish Disposal and the Handling of 'Filth' in Medieval and Early Post-Medieval Towns," in Koen De Groote, Dries Tys, and Marnix Pieters (eds.), *Exchanging Medieval Material Culture: Studies on Archaeology and History Presented to Frans Verhaeghe* (Brussels, 2010): 267–278.
12. Amulree, *Hygienic Conditions*.
13. Evans, "A Good Riddance of Bad Rubbish?"

14. Sheldon Watts, *Epidemics and History: Disease, Power and Imperialism* (New Haven: Yale University Press, 1999), p. 16.
15. Dorothy Porter, *Health, Civilization and the State: A History of Public Health from Ancient to Modern Times* (Abingdon, UK: Routledge, 2005), p. 41.
16. Mark Harrison, *Disease and the Modern World: 1500 to the Present Day* (New York: John Wiley & Sons, 2013), p. 45.
17. Jo Nelson Hays, *The Burdens of Disease: Epidemics and Human Response in Western History* (New Brunswick, NJ: Rutgers University Press, 2009), p. 110.
18. Ibid., p. 165.
19. Simon Szreter, "The Importance of Social Intervention in Britain's Mortality Decline c. 1850–1914: A Re-interpretation of the Role of Public Health," *Social History of Medicine* 1, no. 1 (1988): 1–38.
20. The importance of environment to the disease's impact is suggested by the fact that in the mid-1930s as many as one-third of US college students still tested positive for tuberculosis even though death tolls from the disease were a small fraction of their rate fifty years before. Hays, *The Burdens of Disease*, p. 173.
21. Ibid., pp. 159–162.
22. R. S. Bray, *Armies of Pestilence: The Impact of Disease on History* (Cambridge, UK: James Clarke & Co., 2004), p. 155.
23. Hastings quoted in Watts, *Epidemics and History*, p. 185, and Hays, *The Burdens of Disease*, p. 141.
24. Watts, *Epidemics and History*, p. 167.
25. Bray, *Armies of Pestilence*, p. 162.
26. Hays, *The Burdens of Disease*, p. 135.
27. Porter, *Health, Civilization and the State*, p. 88.
28. Ibid., p. 72.
29. Quoted in Samuel Edward Finer, *The Life and Times of Sir Edwin Chadwick* (Abingdon, UK: Routledge, 2016).
30. Hays, *The Burdens of Disease*, p. 145.
31. Stephen Halliday, "Death and Miasma in Victorian London: An Obstinate Belief," *British Medical Journal* 323, no. 7327 (2001): 1469.
32. Porter, *Health, Civilization and the State*, p. 118.
33. Joseph William Bazalgette, *On the Main Drainage of London: and the Interception of the Sewage from the River Thames* (London: W. Clowes and Sons, 1865).
34. Halliday, *Death and Miasma in Victorian London*.
35. Ibid.
36. Bazalgette, *On the Main Drainage of London*.
37. Ibid., p 14.
38. Gregory Clark, *A Farewell to Alms: A Brief Economic History of the World* (Princeton, NJ: Princeton University Press, 2007), p. 107.
39. Katherine Ashenburg, *The Dirt on Clean* (New York: North Point Press, 2007), p. 102.
40. Ibid., pp. 175 and 233.
41. Szreter, "The Importance of Social Intervention."
42. Fabiana Santana, "The World's Most Expensive Restaurants." Retrieved from http://www.foxnews.com/leisure/2014/12/05/world-most-expensive-restaurants/.

43. Menu retrieved from http://www.thomaskeller.com/sites/default/files/media/4.27.2016_dinner_tasting.pdf.
44. Rande Iaboni, "Posh NYC Restaurant Roasted by Health Inspectors," CNN, March 4, 2014. Retrieved from http://www.cnn.com/2014/03/04/us/new-york-restaurant-health-inspection/.
45. The Council of the City of New York, *Hearing on the Fiscal Year 2014 Executive Budget for the Department of Sanitation*, May 30, 2013. Retrieved from https://council.nyc.gov/budget/wp-content/uploads/sites/54/2013/06/fy2014-deptofsanitation.pdf.
46. New York City, *New York City's Wastewater Treatment System*. Retrieved from https://www.researchgate.net/profile/Rafik_Karaman/post/How_does_government_control_WWTP_effluent/attachment/59d6340879197b8077991b44/AS%3A377579619012609%401467033404974/download/WWTP+NY+USA.pdf.
47. Bureau of Labor Statistics, May 2015, "National Industry-Specific Occupational Employment and Wage Estimates, NAICS 325600—Soap, Cleaning Compound, and Toilet Preparation Manufacturing." Retrieved from https://www.bls.gov/oes/2016/may/naics4_325600.html.
48. Stephan Talty, *The Illustrious Dead: The Terrifying Story of How Typhus Killed Napoleon's Greatest Army* (New York: Crown Publishers, 2009), p. 272.
49. Ibid., p. 273.
50. M. M. Manring et al., "Treatment of War Wounds: A Historical Review," *Clinical Orthopaedics and Related Research* 467, no. 8 (2009): 2168–2191.
51. As late as 1900, four out of ten deaths in the United States were the result of eleven major infectious diseases, chief among them tuberculosis, pneumonia, diphtheria, and typhoid fever. By 1973, only 6 percent of deaths in the US were due to those same causes. But typhoid deaths had fallen from over three per ten thousand people per year in 1900 to negligible levels before the antibiotic chloramphenicol was introduced to fight it in 1948. Tuberculosis was responsible for about two deaths a year for each ten thousand people in the US in 1900. By the time the drug isoniazid was used against tuberculosis in the 1950s, mortality from the disease had fallen by more than three-quarters. Pneumonia mortality rates were a third of their level at the turn of the century by the time that the antibacterial sulfonamide was introduced as a treatment. See John B. McKinlay and Sonja M. McKinlay, "The Questionable Contribution of Medical Measures to the Decline of Mortality in the United States in the Twentieth Century," *Milbank Memorial Fund Quarterly: Health and Society* (1977): 405–428, and Hays, *The Burdens of Disease*, p. 257. That's not to say that vaccines haven't been hugely important to US and European health—between 1924 and 2013, the best estimate is that vaccinations in the US have prevented 103 million cases of polio, measles, rubella, mumps, hepatitis A, diphtheria, and pertussis combined. See van Willem G. Panhuis et al., "Contagious Diseases in the United States from 1888 to the Present," *New England Journal of Medicine* 369, no. 22 (2023): 2152.
52. Hans-Joachim Voth, "Living Standards and the Urban Environment," in *The Cambridge Economic History of Modern Britain* 1: 1700–1860 (2004).

53. Suchit Arora, "Health, Human Productivity and Long-Term Economic Growth," *Journal of Economic History* 61, no. 3 (2001): 699–749.
54. Edward Anthony Wrigley, *Poverty, Progress, and Population* (Cambridge, UK: Cambridge University Press, 2004).
55. Marcella Alsan and Claudia Goldin, *Watersheds in Infant Mortality: The Role of Effective Water and Sewerage Infrastructure, 1880 to 1915*, no. w21263, National Bureau of Economic Research, 2015.
56. As well as other public infrastructure: public transport played a role in extending health gains by reducing housing density. Hays, *The Burdens of Disease*, p.165. Note, however, some evidence of a limited impact of sewage treatment and bacteriological standards for milk in the United States 1900–1940 presented by Anderson et al. These authors suggest better domestic living conditions and nutrition were more significant causes of health improvements (Mark Anderson, Kerwin Kofi Charles, and Daniel Rees, *Public Health Efforts and the Decline in Urban Mortality*, IZA Discussion Paper No. 1773, 2018).
57. Clark, *A Farewell to Alms*, pp. 195 and 283.
58. Myron Echenberg, "Pestis Redux: The Initial Years of the Third Bubonic Plague Pandemic, 1894–1901," *Journal of World History* 13, no. 2 (2002): 429–449.
59. Blaine Harden, "Dr. Matthew's Passion," *New York Times*, February 18, 2001, p. 1.

Chapter Seven: Salvation by Needle

1. Philip C. Grammaticos and Aristidis Diamantis, "Useful Known and Unknown Views of the Father of Modern Medicine, Hippocrates and His Teacher Democritus," *Hellenic Journal of Nuclear Medicine* 11, no. 1 (2008): 2–4.
2. Ibid.
3. Procopius, *History of the Wars, Books I and II*. Retrieved from http://www.gutenberg.org/files/16764/16764-h/16764-h.htm.
4. Reprinted in John Aberth, *The Black Death: The Great Mortality of 1348–1350: A Brief History with Documents* (London: Palgrave Macmillan, 2005), p. 73.
5. Quoted in Aberth *The Black Death*, p. 65.
6. Quoted in Mark Wheelis, "Biological Warfare at the 1346 Siege of Caffa," *Emerging Infectious Diseases* 8, no. 9 (2002): 973.
7. Angela Ki Che Leung, "Organized Medicine in Ming-Qing China: State and Private Medical Institutions in the Lower Yangzi Region," *Late Imperial China* 8, no. 1 (1987): 134–166.
8. Descartes, *Discourse on the Method*. Retrieved from the Project Gutenberg eBook, http://www.gutenberg.org/files/59/59-h/59-h.htm.
9. Monica Rimmer, "How Smallpox Claimed Its Final Victim," BBC News, August 10, 2018, https://www.bbc.com/news/uk-england-birmingham-45101091.
10. Ana T. Duggan, Maria F. Perdomo, Dario Piombino-Mascali, Stephanie Marciniak, Debi Poinar, Matthew V. Emery, Jan P. Buchmann et al., "17th Century Variola Virus Reveals the Recent History of Smallpox," *Current Biology* 26, no. 24 (2016): 3407–3412.

11. Donald R. Hopkins, *The Greatest Killer: Smallpox in History* (Chicago: University of Chicago Press, 2002).
12. Arthur Boylston, "The Origins of Inoculation," *Journal of the Royal Society of Medicine* 105, no. 7 (2012): 309–313.
13. Quoted by Jeanette Farrell, *Invisible Enemies: Stories of Infectious Disease* (New York: Farrar Straus and Giroux, 1998), p. 17.
14. Paul A. David, S. Ryan Johansson, and Andrea Pozzi, *The Demography of an Early Mortality Transition: Life Expectancy, Survival and Mortality Rates for Britain's Royals, 1500–1799*, University of Oxford Discussion Papers in Economic and Social History no. 83, August 2010.
15. Robert Boddice, *Edward Jenner* (Cheltenham, UK: History Press, 2015).
16. Dorothy Crawford, *Deadly Companions: How Microbes Shaped Our History* (Oxford, UK: Oxford University Press, 2007), p. 175.
17. Francesc Asensi-Botet, "Fighting Against Smallpox Around the World: The Vaccination Expedition of Xavier de Balmis (1803–1806) and Josep Salvany (1803–1810)," *Contributions to Science* 8, no. 1(2012): 99–105.
18. Ibid.
19. A. B. Jannetta, *Epidemics and Mortality in Early Modern Japan* (Princeton, NJ: Princeton University Press, 2014).
20. Dorothy Crawford, *Deadly Companions: How Microbes Shaped Our History* (Oxford, UK, Oxford University Press, 2007), p. 175.
21. Jessica Martucci, "Medicinal Leeches and Where to Find Them," Science History Institute blog, March 24, 2020, https://www.sciencehistory.org/distillations/medicinal-leeches-and-where-to-find-them.
22. Farrell, *Invisible Enemies*.
23. Jo Nelson Hays, *The Burdens of Disease: Epidemics and Human Response in Western History* (New Brunswick, NJ: Rutgers University Press, 2009), p. 132.
24. Ibid., p. 141.
25. Ibid., pp. 236–237.
26. Sheryl Persson, *Smallpox, Syphilis and Salvation: Medical Breakthroughs That Changed the World* (Dunedin, NZ: Exisle Publishing, 2010).
27. Ibid.
28. Paul A. Offit, *Vaccinated: One Man's Quest to Defeat the World's Deadliest Diseases* (Washington, DC: Smithsonian Books, 2007).
29. Ibid., pp. 102–3.
30. Ernest Drucker, Phillip G. Alcabes, and Preston A. Marx, "The Injection Century: Massive Unsterile Injections and the Emergence of Human Pathogens," *Lancet* 358, no. 9297 (2001): 1989–1992.
31. Hays, *The Burdens of Disease*, p. 262.
32. Arthur Allen, *The Fantastic Laboratory of Dr. Weigl: How Two Brave Scientists Battled Typhus and Sabotaged the Nazis* (New York: W. W. Norton & Company, 2009).
33. Drucker et al., "The Injection Century" (real dollars in 1998 USD).
34. Ibid.
35. Jacques Pepin et al., "Evolution of the Global Burden of Viral Infections from Unsafe Medical Injections, 2000–2010," *PloS One* 9, no. 6 (2014).
36. Quoted by Crawford, *Deadly Companions*, p. 176.

37. Donald R. Hopkins, *The Greatest Killer: Smallpox in History* (Chicago: University of Chicago Press, 2002), p. 305.
38. Donald Henderson, "Eradication: Lessons from the Past," MMWR, December 31, 1999, 48:16–22. Retrieved from http://www.cdc.gov/MMWR/preview/mmwrhtml/su48a6.htm.
39. Crawford, *Deadly Companions*, p. 222.
40. Polio Global Eradication Initiative, "Remembering Ali Maalin," http://polioeradication.org/news-post/remembering-ali-maalin/.
41. Source: the World Health Organization database. Retrieved from http://www.who.int/gho/database/en/.
42. Data from the Polio Global Eradication Initiative: http://www.polioeradication.org/dataandmonitoring/poliothisweek.aspx.
43. Vaccines list from the Centers for Disease Control, https://www.cdc.gov/vaccines/vpd/vaccines-list.html.
44. James C. Riley, *Rising Life Expectancy: A Global History* (Cambridge, UK: Cambridge University Press, 2001).
45. World Health Organization, "Miracle Cure for an Old Scourge: An Interview with Dr. Dilip Mahalanabis," http://www.who.int/bulletin/volumes/87/2/09-060209/en/, and Sumati Yengkhom, "Global Glory, but State Apathy for ORS Creator," *Times of India* May 13, 2013, http://timesofindia.indiatimes.com/city/kolkata/Global-glory-but-state-apathy-for-ORS-creator/articleshow/20022013.cms.
46. Olivier Fontaine and Charlotte Newton, "A Revolution in the Management of Diarrhoea," *Bulletin of the World Health Organization* 79, no. 5 (2001): 471–472.
47. Val Curtis and Sandy Cairncross, "Effect of Washing Hands with Soap on Diarrhoea Risk in the Community: A Systematic Review," *Lancet Infectious Diseases*, no. 3 (2003): 275–281.
48. Rosemary Drisdelle, *Parasites: Tales of Humanity's Most Unwelcome Guests* (Berkeley: University of of California Press, 2010).
49. Aaron Carroll, "Lessons from the Low-Tech Defeat of Guinea Worm," *New York Times*, August 12, 2014 http://www.nytimes.com/2014/08/12/upshot/lessons-from-the-low-tech-defeat-of-the-guinea-worm-.html.
50. Pinar Mine Güneş, "The Role of Maternal Education in Child Health: Evidence from a Compulsory Schooling Law," *Economics of Education Review* 47 (2015): 1–16.
51. Source: World Bank data, https://data.worldbank.org/indicator/SH.STA.BASS.ZS?end=2015&start=2000.
52. Sonia Bhalotra et al., *Urban Water Disinfection and Mortality Decline in Developing Countries*, University of Essex Institute for Social and Economic Research Working Paper 2017-04.
53. Peter Katona and Judit Katona-Apte, "The Interaction Between Nutrition and Infection," *Clinical Infectious Diseases* 46, no. 10 (2008): 1582–1588, and Our World in Data https://ourworldindata.org/food-per-person.
54. Cecilia Tacoli, Gordon McGranahan, and David Satterthwaite, "Urbanization, Poverty and Inequity: Is Rural-Urban Migration a Poverty Problem or Part of the Solution," *The New Global Frontier: Urbanization, Poverty and Environment in the 21st Century* (2008): 37–53, updated with Goufrane Mansour et al., "Situation Analysis

of the Urban Sanitation Sector in Kenya," 2017, https://www.wsup.com/content/uploads/2017/09/Situation-analysis-of-the-urban-sanitation-sector-in-Kenya.pdf.

55. Charles Kenny, *Getting Better: Why Global Development Is Succeeding—and How We Can Improve the World Even More* (New York: Basic Books, 2012). Maryaline Catillon, David Cutler, and Thomas Getzen, *Two Hundred Years of Health and Medical Care: The Importance of Medical Care for Life Expectancy Gains*, no. w25330, National Bureau of Economic Research, 2018, report that doctors made up 0.8 percent of the US workforce in 1850 and 0.3 percent in 1950—that decline took place during a period of massively improving health (as well as standards among medical practitioners, of course).
56. Rodrigo R. Soares, "On the Determinants of Mortality Reductions in the Developing World," *Population and Development Review* 33, no. 2 (2007): 247–287.
57. Because infection as a killer skews young, it accounts for a higher proportion of years of life potential lost, but even according to that measure we crossed the line into a greater burden of disease from noncommunicable disease toward the end of last century. In 2000, the World Health Organization estimates that 43 percent of life years were lost to communicable disease. By 2012, that had dropped to around one-third. WHO estimates for 2000–2012 disease burden from http://www.who.int/healthinfo/global_burden_disease/estimates/en/index2.html.
58. John B. McKinlay and Sonja M. McKinlay, "The Questionable Contribution of Medical Measures to the Decline of Mortality in the United States in the Twentieth Century," *Milbank Memorial Fund Quarterly: Health and Society* (1977): 405–428.
59. Alberto Palloni and Randy Wyrick, "Mortality Decline in Latin America: Changes in the Structure of Causes of Deaths, 1950–1975," *Social Biology* 28, nos. 3–4 (1981): 187–216.
60. Rafael Lozano et al., "Global and Regional Mortality from 235 Causes of Death for 20 Age Groups in 1990 and 2010: A Systematic Analysis for the Global Burden of Disease Study 2010," *Lancet* 380, no. 9859 (2013): 2095–2128. I calculate infectious diseases as communicable, maternal, neonatal, and nutritional deaths (Group One), subtracting all maternal, neonatal, and nutritional deaths apart from those attributable to sepsis.
61. Under-five mortality data from www.gapminder.org.
62. Yvonne Lefèber and Henk W. A. Voorhoeve, *Indigenous Customs in Childbirth and Child Care* (Assen, Netherlands: Uitgeverij Van Gorcum, 1998).
63. Peter N. Stearns, *Childhood in World History* (Abingdon, UK: Routledge, 2010).
64. Bill Gates, "Why Naming a Child Is a Revolutionary Act," *Impatient Optimists* blog http://www.impatientoptimists.org/Posts/2013/02/Why-Is-Naming-a-Child-a-Revolutionary-Act.
65. Max Roser, *Life Expectancy* (OurWorldInData.org, 2016). Retrieved from http://ourworldindata.org/data/population-growth-vital-statistics/life-expectancy/.
66. Sources for 2016 GDP PPP per capita, poverty, and life expectancy are the World Bank's World Development Indicators (https://data.worldbank.org/) and PovcalNet (http://iresearch.worldbank.org/PovcalNet/povOnDemand.aspx). For England and Wales life expectancy, UK Office of National Statistics (https://www.ons.gov.uk/peoplepopulationandcommunity/birthsdeathsandmarriages/lifeex

pectancies/articles/howhaslifeexpectancychangedovertime/2015-09-09) and UK GDP PPP per capita, the MaddisonProject website (https://www.rug.nl/ggdc/historicaldevelopment/maddison/releases/maddison-project-database-2018).

67. Shiyon Wang, P. Marquez, and John Langenbrunner, "Toward a Healthy and Harmonious Life in China: Stemming the Rising Tide of Non-Communicable Diseases," mimeo, the World Bank, 2011.
68. Elizabeth Frankenberg, Jessica Y. Ho, and Duncan Thomas, *Biological Health Risks and Economic Development*, no. w21277, National Bureau of Economic Research, 2015.
69. Adult obesity data from the Harvard School of Public Health, http://www.hsph.harvard.edu/obesity-prevention-source/obesity-trends/obesity-rates-worldwide/.
70. World Food Program statistics on hunger: http://www.wfp.org/hunger/stats. For an extended discussion of the growth of the noninfectious disease threats, see Thomas J. Bollyky, *Plagues and the Paradox of Progress: Why the World Is Getting Healthier in Worrisome Ways* (Cambridge, MA: MIT Press, 2018).

Chapter Eight: It's Good to Get Closer

1. Sheldon Watts, *Epidemics and History: Disease, Power and Imperialism* (New Haven: Yale University Press, 1999), p. 262.
2. Nathan Nunn and Nancy Qian, "The Columbian Exchange: A History of Disease, Food, and Ideas," *Journal of Economic Perspectives* 24, no. 2 (2010): 163–188.
3. Jeanette Farrell, *Invisible Enemies: Stories of Infectious Disease* (New York: Farrar Straus and Giroux, 1998), pp. 154–158.
4. Watts, *Epidemics and History*, p. 258.
5. Michael B. A. Oldstone, *Viruses, Plagues, and History: Past, Present, and Future* (Oxford, UK: Oxford University Press. 2009), p. 123.
6. Frederick Fox Cartwright and Michael Denis Biddiss, *Disease and History* (New York: Marboro Books, 1972), p. 164.
7. Watts, *Epidemics and History*, p. 258.
8. Jo Nelson Hays, *The Burdens of Disease: Epidemics and Human Response in Western History* (New Brunswick, NJ: Rutgers University Press, 2009), pp. 206–210.
9. Andrew Spielman and Michael d'Antonio, *Mosquito: The Story of Man's Deadliest Foe* (New York: Hyperion, 2002), p. 126.
10. Marcella Alsan, "The Effect of the Tsetse Fly on African Development," *American Economic Review* 105, no. 1 (2015): 382–410.
11. Quoted in Rosemary Drisdelle, *Parasites: Tales of Humanity's Most Unwelcome Guests* (Berkeley: University of California Press, 2010), p. 18.
12. Watts, *Epidemics and History*, p. 266.
13. Mark Harrison, *Disease and the Modern World: 1500 to the Present Day* (New York: John Wiley & Sons, 2013).
14. Abhijit V. Banerjee and Esther Duflo "The Economic Lives of the Poor," *Journal of Economic Perspectives* 21, no. 1 (2007): 141.
15. Data compiled by the Yale University SETO lab, http://urban.yale.edu/data, and

the UN Department of Economic and Social Affairs, https://esa.un.org/unpd/wup/CD-ROM/.

16. Edward Glaeser and David Maré, "Cities and Skills," *Journal of Labor Economics* 19, no. 2 (2001): 316–342.
17. R. Dobbs et al., *Urban World: Mapping the Economic Power of Cities* (McKinsey Global Institute, 2011).
18. Charles Kenny, "Cheer Up Liberals," *Businessweek*, November 3, 2014, http://www.businessweek.com/articles/2014-11-03/cheer-up-liberals-city-dwellers-will-soon-rule-the-world.
19. See, for example, Alice Evans and Liam Swiss, "Why Do Cities Tend to Disrupt Gender Ideologies and Inequalities?" mimeo, Cambridge University, 2017.
20. Stephen W. Hargarten and S. P. Baker, "Fatalities in the Peace Corps, A Retrospective Study: 1962 Through 1983," *Journal of the American Medical Association* 254 (1985): 1326–1329. See also Prakash Bhatta, P. Simkhada, E. Van Teijlingen, and S. Maybin, "A Questionnaire Study of Voluntary Service Overseas (VSO) Volunteers: Health Risk and Problems Encountered," *Journal of Travel Medicine* 16, no. 5 (2009): 332–337.
21. Julie Y. Huang, Alexandra Sedlovskaya, Joshua M. Ackerman, and John A. Bargh, "Immunizing Against Prejudice: Effects of Disease Protection on Attitudes Toward Out-Groups," *Psychological Science* 22, no. 12 (2011): 1550–1556.
22. B. Dupont, A. Gandhi, and T. J. Weiss, *The American Invasion of Europe: The Long Term Rise in Overseas Travel, 1820–2000*, no. w13977, National Bureau of Economic Research, 2008.
23. Data source: World Bank Databank, https://databank.worldbank.org/home.aspx.
24. New America Economy Research Fund, "Immigrant Healthcare Workers Are Critical in the Fight Against Covid-19," https://research.newamericaneconomy.org/report/covid-19-immigrant-healthcare-workers/.
25. Data from Starbucks (http://www.starbucks.com/business/international-stores) and OECD statistics (https://data.oecd.org/fdi/fdi-stocks.htm).
26. Angus Maddison, "The West and the Rest in the World Economy: 1000–2030," *World Economics* 9, no. 4 (2008): 75–99.
27. Charles Kenny, *The Upside of Down: Why the Rise of the Rest Is Good for the West* (New York: Basic Books, 2014).
28. Chad Bown, "COVID-19: Trump's Curbs on Exports of Medical Gear Put Americans and Others at Risk," Peterson Institute for International Economics blog, https://www.piie.com/blogs/trade-and-investment-policy-watch/covid-19-trumps-curbs-exports-medical-gear-put-americans-and.
29. US Geological Survey, "Cobalt Statistics and Information," http://minerals.usgs.gov/minerals/pubs/commodity/cobalt/mcs-2016-cobal.pdf.
30. World Health Organization, *The World Medicines Situation* (Geneva: World Health Organization, 2004).
31. Helen Branswell, "Against All Odds," *STAT*, January 7, 2020, https://www.statnews.com/2020/01/07/inside-story-scientists-produced-world-first-ebola-vaccine/.
32. Charles I. Jones and Paul M. Romer, "The New Kaldor Facts: Ideas, Institutions, Population, and Human Capital," *American Economic Journal: Macroeconomics* 2, no. 1 (2010): 224–245.

33. Luis Angeles, "Demographic Transitions: Analyzing the Effects of Mortality on Fertility," *Journal of Population Economics* 23, no. 1 (2010): 99–120.
34. David Roodman, "The Impact of Life Saving Interventions on Fertility," *David Roodman* blog, April 16, 2014, http://davidroodman.com/blog/2014/04/16/the-mortality-fertility-link/.
35. David E. Bloom and David Canning, *Global Demographic Change: Dimensions and Economic Significance*, no. w10817, National Bureau of Economic Research, 2004.
36. Stefania Albanesi and Claudia Olivetti, *Gender Roles and Medical Progress*, no. w14873, National Bureau of Economic Research, 2009.
37. Mark Schaller and Damian Murray, "Infectious Disease and the Creation of Culture," *Advances in Culture and Psychology* 1 (2011).
38. Charles Kenny and Dev Patel, *Norms and Reform: Legalizing Homosexuality Improves Attitudes*, CGD Working Paper 465, Center for Global Development, Washington, DC, 2017.
39. Daniel Cohen and Laura Leker, *Health and Education: Another Look with the Proper Data*, no. 9940, CEPR Discussion Papers, 2014; see also Casper Worm Hansen, *The Effect of Life Expectancy on Schooling: Evidence from the International Health Transition*, Discussion Papers of Business and Economics, University of Southern Denmark, 2012.
40. Sebnem Kalemli-Ozcan, "AIDS Reversal of the Demographic Transition and Economic Development: Evidence from Africa," *Journal of Population Economics* 25, no. 3 (2012): 871–897.
41. Emily Oster, "HIV and Sexual Behavior Change: Why Not Africa?" *Journal of Health Economics* 31, no. 1 (2012): 35–49.
42. Steven Pinker, *Enlightenment Now: The Case for Reason, Science, Humanism, and Progress* (New York: Viking, 2018), pp. 159–161. Azar Gat, a professor of national security at Tel Aviv University, examined the relationship between the decline of war and the process of modernization and suggested it involved a number of interacting elements. These included the escape from Malthusianism, economic development, commercial interdependence, growing risk aversion, urbanism, liberal attitudes including those toward sexual freedom, aging demographics, and the changing role of women. We have seen all of these factors are in turn linked to declining infection (Azar Gat, *The Causes of War and the Spread of Peace: But Will War Rebound?* [Oxford, UK: Oxford University Press, 2017], Chapter 6.)
43. Dean T. Jamison et al., "Global Health 2035: A World Converging Within a Generation," *Lancet* 382, no. 9908 (2013): 1898–1955, and Jeffrey Sachs and Pia Malaney, "The Economic and Social Burden of Malaria," *Nature* 415, no. 6872 (2002): 680–685.
44. See William Easterly and Ross Levine, "Tropics, Germs, and Crops: How Endowments Influence Economic Development," *Journal of Monetary Economics* 50, no. 1 (2003): 3–39, on the relative contribution.
45. Philippe Aghion, Peter Howitt, and Fabrice Murtin, *The Relationship Between Health and Growth: When Lucas Meets Nelson-Phelps*, no. w15813, National Bureau of Economic Research, 2010; see also Suchit Arora, "Health, Human Productivity, and Long-Term Economic Growth," *Journal of Economic History* 61, no. 3 (2001): 699–749.

46. Sourced from the Maddison Project website, https://www.rug.nl/ggdc/historical development/maddison/releases/maddison-project-database-2018.
47. Data from the original Angus Maddison database, https://www.rug.nl/ggdc/his toricaldevelopment/maddison/?lang=en.

Chapter Nine: The Revenge of Infection?

1. Lisa Benton-Short, M. D. Price, and S. Friedman, "Globalization from Below: The Ranking of Global Immigrant Cities," *International Journal of Urban and Regional Research* 29, no. 4 (2005): 945–959.
2. Burnet noted the risk of emergent diseases but predicted "they will presumably be safely maintained." Macfarlane Burnet and David White, *Natural History of Infectious Disease* (Cambridge, UK: Cambridge University Press, 1972), p. 263.
3. CDC MMWR, June 5, 1981 / 30(21): 1–3, http://www.cdc.gov/mmwr/preview /mmwrhtml/june_5.htm.
4. Faria et al., "The Early Spread and Epidemic Ignition of HIV-1 in Human Populations," *Science* 346, no. 6205 (2014): 56–61.
5. David Serwadda et al., "Slim Disease: A New Disease in Uganda and Its Association with HTLV-III Infection," *Lancet* 326, no. 8460 (1985): 849–852.
6. J. Steinberg, "AIDS Prevention Is Thicker Than Blood. Zimbabwe," *Links* 9, no. 2 (1992): 3–3.
7. Emily Oster, "Routes of Infection: Exports and HIV Incidence in Sub-Saharan Africa," *Journal of the European Economic Association* 10, no. 5 (2012): 1025–1058.
8. Jim Todd et al., "Editorial: Measuring HIV-Related Mortality in the First Decade of Anti-Retroviral Therapy in Sub-Saharan Africa," *Global Health Action* 7 (May 2014).
9. World Health Organization data on number of deaths due to HIV/AIDS, http:// www.who.int/gho/hiv/epidemic_status/deaths_text/en/.
10. Katherine F. Smith et al., "Global Rise in Infectious Disease Outbreaks," *Journal of the Royal Society Interface* 6, no. 11 (2014).
11. David M. Morens, Gregory K. Folkers, and Anthony S. Fauci, "Emerging Infections: A Perpetual Challenge," *Lancet Infectious Diseases* 8, no. 11 (2008): 710–719.
12. David M. Morens, Gregory K. Folkers, and Anthony S. Fauci, "The Challenge of Emerging and Re-emerging Infectious Diseases," *Nature* 430, no. 6996 (2004): 242–249, and CDC information on Nipa, http://www.cdc.gov/vhf/nipah/symp toms/index.html.
13. Dorothy Crawford, *The Invisible Enemy: A Natural History of Viruses* (Oxford, UK: Oxford University Press, 2000), p. 34.
14. Benjamin L. Hart, "Behavioral Adaptations to Pathogens and Parasites: Five Strategies," *Neuroscience & Biobehavioral Reviews* 14, no. 3 (1990): 273–294.
15. See also Robert De Vries et al., "Three Mutations Switch H7N9 Influenza to Human-Type Receptor Specificity," *PLoS Pathogens* 13, no. 6 (2017). A final source of new infectious challenges is the recognition that old diseases considered noninfectious sometimes have an infection as a cause—liver cancer caused by

hepatitis B, ulcers caused by *Helicobacter pylori*, and cervical cancer caused by human papillomavirus, for example.

16. CDC MMWR Weekly, April 24, 2009, 58/15, "Swine Influenza A (H1N1) Infection in Two Children—Southern California, March–April 2009." Retrieved from http://www.cdc.gov/mmwr/preview/mmwrhtml/mm5815a5.htm.
17. CDC MMWR Weekly, May 8, 2009, 58/17, "Update: Novel Influenza A (H1N1) Virus Infections—Worldwide, May 6, 2009." Retrieved from http://www.cdc.gov/mmwr/preview/mmwrhtml/mm5817a1.htm.
18. Sundar S. Shrestha et al., "Estimating the Burden of 2009 Pandemic Influenza A (H1N1) in the United States (April 2009–April 2010)," *Clinical Infectious Diseases* 52, suppl. 1 (2011): S75–S82.
19. FAOStat data from http://www.fao.org/faostat/en/#data/QL.
20. Kimberly Elliott, *Feeding the Future or Favoring American Farmers* (Washington, DC: Brookings, 2016).
21. David Tilman et al., "Agricultural Sustainability and Intensive Production Practices," *Nature* 418, no. 6898 (2002): 671–677.
22. Michaeleen Doucleff and Jane Greenhalgh, "A Taste for Pork Helped a Deadly Virus Jump to Humans," *Goats and Soda*, NPR, February 25, 2017, https://www.npr.org/sections/goatsandsoda/2017/02/25/515258818/a-taste-for-pork-helped-a-deadly-virus-jump-to-humans.
23. FAOStat data from http://www.fao.org/faostat/en/#data/QL.
24. Joyce Dargay, Dermot Gately, and Martin Sommer, "Vehicle Ownership and Income Growth, Worldwide: 1960–2030," *Energy Journal* (2007): 143–170.
25. Andrew J. Tatem, David J. Rogers, and S. I. Hay, "Global Transport Networks and Infectious Disease Spread," *Advances in Parasitology* 62 (2006): 293–343.
26. Dorothy Crawford, *Deadly Companions: How Microbes Shaped Our History* (Oxford, UK: Oxford University Press, 2007), pp. 5–6.
27. Tatem et al., "Global Transport Networks."
28. Our World in Data, Coronavius, https://ourworldindata.org/coronavirus.
29. Ronald Barrett et al., "Emerging and Re-emerging Infectious Diseases: The Third Epidemiologic Transition," *Annual Review of Anthropology* (1998): 247–271.
30. Gillian K. SteelFisher, Robert J. Blendon, and Narayani Lasala-Blanco, "Ebola in the United States—Public Reactions and Implications," *New England Journal of Medicine* 373, no. 9 (2015): 789–791.
31. Casey B. Mulligan, *Economic Activity and the Value of Medical Innovation During a Pandemic*, University of Chicago, Becker Friedman Institute for Economics Working Paper 2020-48, 2020.
32. Paolo Bajardi et al., "Human Mobility Networks, Travel Restrictions, and the Global Spread of 2009 H1N1 Pandemic," *PLoS ONE* 6, no. 1 (2011).
33. Council on Foreign Relations (2020), *Tracking Coronavirus in Countries With and Without Travel Bans*, https://www.thinkglobalhealth.org/article/tracking-coronavirus-countries-and-without-travel-bans.
34. Alex Nowrasteh and Andrew Forrester, *How US Travel Restrictions on China Affected the Spread of Covid-19 in the United States*, Cato Working Paper no. 58, 2020.
35. Principles for Responsible Investment, "CES Convention May Have Spread Coronavirus Throughout the US—and World," April 24, 2020, https://www.pri.org

/stories/2020-04-24/ces-convention-may-have-spread-coronavirus-throughout-us-and-world.

36. "2 Californians Died of Coronavirus Weeks Before Previously Known 1st US Death," CNN, April 22, 2020, https://www.cnn.com/2020/04/22/us/california-deaths-earliest-in-us/index.html.
37. Steve Eder et al., "430,000 People Have Traveled from China to U.S. Since Coronavirus Surfaced," *New York Times*, April 4, 2020, https://www.nytimes.com/2020/04/04/us/coronavirus-china-travel-restrictions.html.
38. David Bier, "US Airports Had 10.7 Million Entries from Countries with Covid-19 Cases," *Cato* blog, https://www.cato.org/blog/us-airports-had-107-million-entries-nations-covid-19.
39. Doug Saunders, "Why Travel Bans Fail to Stop Pandemics," *Foreign Affairs*, May 15, 2020, https://www.foreignaffairs.com/articles/canada/2020-05-15/why-travel-bans-fail-stop-pandemics.
40. From the Council on Foreign Relations global list of travel bans: https://www.thinkglobalhealth.org/article/travel-restrictions-china-due-covid-19.
41. Julia Hollingsworth, "How New Zealand 'Eliminated' Covid-19," CNN, April 28, 2020, https://www.cnn.com/2020/04/28/asia/new-zealand-coronavirus-outbreak-elimination-intl-hnk/index.html.
42. Joseph Amon and Katherine Todrys, "Fear of Foreigners: HIV-Related Restrictions on Entry, Stay, and Residence," *Journal of the International AIDS Society* 11, no. 1 (2008): 8.
43. Tatem et al., "Global Transport Networks."
44. Commission on a Global Health Risk Framework for the Future, National Academy of Medicine, Secretariat, *The Neglected Dimension of Global Security: A Framework to Counter Infectious Disease Crises*, (National Academy of Medicine, 2015) http://www.nap.edu/catalog/21891/the-neglected-dimension-of-global-security-a-framework-to-counter.
45. Davide Furceri, Prakash Loungani, Jonathan D. Ostry, and Pietro Pizzuto, "Will Covid-19 Affect Inequality? Evidence from Past Pandemics," *Covid Economics* 12 (2020): 138–157.
46. CDC map of US plague locations, http://www.cdc.gov/plague/maps/.

Chapter Ten: Abusing Our Best Defenses

1. McNeil et al., "How a Medical Mystery in Brazil Led Doctors to Zika," *New York Times*, February 7, 2016, http://www.nytimes.com/2016/02/07/health/zika-virus-brazil-how-it-spread-explained.html.
2. Julia Belluz, "Zero: The Number of New Zika Cases from the Rio Olympics," *Vox*, September 3, 2016, http://www.vox.com/2016/9/3/12774610/numer-zika-cases-olympics.
3. Jon Cohen, "Zika Has All But Disappeared in the Americas. Why?" *Science*, August 16, 2017, http://www.sciencemag.org/news/2017/08/zika-has-all-disappeared-americas-why.
4. R. Lourenço-de-Oliveira et al., "*Aedes aegypti* in Brazil: Genetically Differenti-

ated Populations with High Susceptibility to Dengue and Yellow Fever Viruses," *Transactions of the Royal Society of Tropical Medicine and Hygiene* 98, no. 1 (2004): 43–54.

5. Maria de Lourdes G. Macoris et al., "Resistance of *Aedes aegypti* from the State of São Paulo, Brazil, to Organophosphates Insecticides," *Memórias do Instituto Oswaldo Cruz* 98, no. 5 (2003): 703–708.
6. Global Burden of Disease data from http://www.healthmetricsandevaluation.org/gbd/visualizations/gbd-cause-patterns. The low number is produced by adding HIV/AIDS and tuberculoisis, diarrhea, LRI, other infections, NTD, and malaria, along with the category "other communicable diseases." The high number adds neonatal disorders and nutritional deficiencies.
7. World Health Organization data, http://www.who.int/healthinfo/global_burden_disease/estimates/en/index1.html. I calculate infectious diseases as communicable, maternal, neonatal, and nutritional deaths (Group One), subtracting all maternal, neonatal, and nutritional deaths apart from those attributable to sepsis.
8. World Health Organization global immunization data, http://www.who.int/immunization/monitoring_surveillance/global_immunization_data.pdf.
9. Data from WHO/UNICEF Joint Monitoring Report on Drinking Water and Sanitation, http://www.unwater.org/publications/jmp/en/.
10. This is about changing behaviors, which can be deeply ingrained and culturally determined. Michael Geruso and Dean Spears, *Sanitation and Health Externalities: Resolving the Muslim Mortality Paradox*, University of Texas at Austin Working Paper, 2014.
11. Dorothy Porter and Roy Porter, "The Politics of Prevention: Anti-Vaccinationism and Public Health in Nineteenth-Century England," *Medical History* 32, no. 3 (1988): 244.
12. D. Trambaiolo, "Vaccination and the Politics of Medical Knowledge in Nineteenth-Century Japan," *Bulletin of the History of Medicine* 88, no. 3 (2014): 431–456.
13. Mahatma Gandhi, *A Guide to Health* (Aukland, NZ: The Floating Press, 2014).
14. Mark Harrison, *Disease and the Modern World: 1500 to the Present Day* (New York: John Wiley & Sons, 2013).
15. BBC News, "Swansea Measles Epidemic: Worries over MMR Uptake After Outbreak," June 10, 2013, http://www.bbc.co.uk/news/uk-wales-politics-23244628.
16. Paul A. Offit, *Vaccinated: One Man's Quest to Defeat the World's Deadliest Diseases* (Washington, DC: Smithsonian Books, 2007), pp. 159–168.
17. Olga Khazan, "Wealthy LA Schools' Vaccination Rates Are as Low as South Sudan's," *The Atlantic*, September 16, 2004, http://www.theatlantic.com/health/archive/2014/09/wealthy-la-schools-vaccination-rates-are-as-low-as-south-sudans/380252/.
18. Varun Phadke et al., "Association Between Vaccine Refusal and Vaccine-Preventable Diseases in the United States: A Review of Measles and Pertussis," *JAMA* 315, no. 11 (2016): 1149–1158.
19. Seth Mnookin, "The Return of Measles," *Boston Globe*, September 28, 2013, http://www.bostonglobe.com/magazine/2013/09/28/true-cost-not-vaccinating-the-return-measles/4PBenymtmf0CE9WOT1FUWI/story.html.

20. Quoted in Peter Lipson, "Anti-Vaccine Doctors Should Lose Their Licences," *Forbes*, January 30, 2015.
21. H. J. Larson et al., "The State of Vaccine Confidence 2016: Global Insights Through a 67-Country Survey," *EBioMedicine* 12 (2016): 295–301.
22. Alex Kemper, Matthew Davis, and Gary Freed, "Expected Adverse Events in a Mass Smallpox Vaccination Campaign," *Effective Clinical Practice* 5 (2002): 84–90.
23. BBC News, "Kano Shuns Nigeria Polio Campaign," December 12, 2003, http://news.bbc.co.uk/2/hi/africa/3313419.stm.
24. BBC News, "White House: CIA Has Ended Use of Vaccine Programmes," May 20, 2014, http://www.bbc.com/news/world-us-canada-27489045.
25. "Pakistan Polio Vaccinator's Murder by Militants Raises Health Workers' Fears," *Guardian*, March 25, 2014, http://www.theguardian.com/society/2014/mar/25/pakistan-polo-vaccinators-murder-militants-salma-farooqi.
26. Edgar Chavez et al., *Eradicating Polio in Afghanistan and Pakistan*, mimeo, Center for Strategic and International Studies, 2012.
27. Susan V. Lynch et al., "Effects of Early-Life Exposure to Allergens and Bacteria on Recurrent Wheeze and Atopy in Urban Children," *Journal of Allergy and Clinical Immunology* 134, no. 3 (2014): 593–601.
28. E. M. Rees Clayton, M. Todd, J. B. Dowd, and A. Aiello, "The Impact of Bisphenol A and Triclosan on Immune Parameters in the U.S. Population, NHANES 2003–2006," *Environmental Health Perspectives* 119, no. 3 (2011): 390–396.
29. Katri Korpela et al., "Intestinal Microbiome Is Related to Lifetime Antibiotic Use in Finnish Pre-School Children," *Nature Communications* 7 (2016).
30. Eisenhower's State of the Union Address. Retrieved from http://www.pbs.org/wgbh/americanexperience/features/primary-resources/eisenhower-state58/.
31. Andrew Spielman and Michael d'Antonio, *Mosquito: The Story of Man's Deadliest Foe* (New York: Hyperion, 2002).
32. Rosemary Drisdelle, *Parasites: Tales of Humanity's Most Unwelcome Guests* (Berkeley: University of California Press, 2010).
33. Richard G. A. Feachem et al., "Shrinking the Malaria Map: Progress and Prospects," *Lancet* 376, no. 9752 (2010): 1566–1578.
34. Shallo Daba Hamusse, Taye T. Balcha, and Tefera Belachew, "The Impact of Indoor Residual Spraying on Malaria Incidence in East Shoa Zone, Ethiopia," *Global Health Action* 5 (2012).
35. There is the related issue of low-quality drugs. Around 30 percent of the world's public authorities have no drug regulation capacity or a capacity that barely functions. Gaurvika M. L. Nayyar et al., "Poor-Quality Antimalarial Drugs in Southeast Asia and Sub-Saharan Africa," *Lancet Infectious Diseases* 12, no. 6 (2012): 488–496.
36. World Health Organization, *Antimicrobial Resistance: Global Report on Surveillance*, (Geneva: WHO, 2014) http://www.who.int/drugresistance/documents/surveillancereport/en/.
37. Dean T. Jamison et al. (eds.), *Disease Control Priorities in Developing Countries* (Washington, DC: World Bank, 2006).

38. Rachel Nugent, Emma Back, and Alexandra Beith, *The Race Against Drug Resistance* (Washington, DC: Center for Global Development, 2010).
39. Fleming's Nobel Prize acceptance speech. Retrieved from https://www.nobelprize.org/uploads/2018/06/fleming-lecture.pdf.
40. CDC typhoid fever FAQ, http://www.cdc.gov/ncidod/dbmd/diseaseinfo/files/typhoid_fever_FAQ.pdf.
41. E. S. Anderson, "The Problem and Implications of Chloramphenicol Resistance in the Typhoid Bacillus," *Journal of Hygiene* 74, no. 2 (1975): 289–299.
42. Michael L. Barnett and Jeffrey A. Linder, "Antibiotic Prescribing to Adults with Sore Throat in the United States, 1997–2010," *JAMA Internal Medicine* 174, no. 1 (2014): 138–140.
43. The O'Niell Review, *Safe, Secure and Controlled: Managing the Supply Chain of Antimicrobials. The Review on Antimicrobial Resistance Chaired by Jim O'Niell*, November 2015, https://amr-review.org/Publications.html.
44. Christina Larson, "How China Tackled the Risky Over-Prescription of Antibiotics," *Businessweek*, December 6, 2013, http://www.businessweek.com/articles/2013-12-06/how-china-tackled-the-risky-overprescription-of-antibiotics.
45. Ganchimeg Togoobaatar et al., "Survey of Non-Prescribed Use of Antibiotics for Children in an Urban Community in Mongolia," *Bulletin of the World Health Organization* 88, no. 12 (2010): 930–936.
46. Congressional testimony of Stuart Levy in 2010. Retrieved from http://www.tufts.edu/med/apua/policy/7.14.10.pdf.
47. FDA, *Annual Summary Report on Antimicrobials Sold or Distributed in 2013 for Use in Food-Producing Animals*, 2013. Retrieved from https://www.fda.gov/animal-veterinary/news-events/cvm-updates.
48. Kimberly Elliott, *Feeding the Future or Favoring American Farmers* (Washington, DC: Brookings, 2016).
49. FDA National Antimicrobial Resistance Monitoring System, 2011 Report. Retrieved from http://www.fda.gov/downloads/AnimalVeterinary/SafetyHealth/AntimicrobialResistance/NationalAntimicrobialResistanceMonitoringSystem/UCM334834.pdf.
50. FDA press release, "FDA Releases 2012 and 2013 NARMS Integrated Annual Report." Retrieved from https://www.fda.gov/animal-veterinary/news-events/cvm-updates.
51. James Gallagher, "Antibiotic Resistance: World on Cusp of 'Post-Antibiotic Era,'" *BBC News*, November 19, 2015, http://www.bbc.com/news/health-34857015.
52. Victoria Fan and Rifaiyat Mahbub, "US Move on Livestock Antibiotics Includes Possibly Fatal Loophole," *CGD* blog, https://www.cgdev.org/blog/us-move-livestock-antibiotics-includes-possibly-fatal-loophole.
53. World Health Organization, *Antimicrobial Resistance: Global Report on Surveillance* (Geneva: World Health Organization, 2014).
54. Ryan McNeill, Deborah Nelson, and Yasmeen Abutaleb, "Suberbug Scourge Spreads as US Fails to Track Rising Human Toll," Reuters.com, September 7, 2016.
55. Beth Mole, "MRSA: Farming Up Trouble," *Nature*, July 24, 2013, http://www.nature.com/news/mrsa-farming-up-trouble-1.13427.

56. The Review on Antimicrobial Resistance, *Antimicrobial Resistance: Tackling a Crisis* (2014). Retrieved from https://amr-review.org/Publications.html.
57. Ibid.
58. CDC press brefing transcript from September 16, 2016, http://www.cdc.gov/media/releases/2013/t0916_health-threats.html.
59. Sara Cosgrove and Yehuda Carmeli, "The Impact of Antimicrobial Resistance on Health and Economic Outcomes," *Antimicribial Resistance* 36 (2003): 1433.
60. The Review on Antimicrobial Resistance, *Antimicrobial Resistance.*
61. Burden of Disease data retrieved from http://www.healthmetricsandevaluation.org/gbd/visualizations/gbd-cause-patterns and WHO, *Quantitative Risk Assessment of the Effects of Climate Change on Selected Causes of Death, 2030s and 2050s* (Geneva: World Health Organization, 2014), http://apps.who.int/iris/bitstream/10665/134014/1/9789241507691_eng.pdf.
62. The Global Terrorism Index 2014. Retrieved from http://www.visionofhumanity.org/sites/default/files/Global%20Terrorism%20Index%20Report%202014_0.pdf.
63. CDC, *Antibiotic Threats in the United States, 2013*, http://www.cdc.gov/drugresistance/threat-report-2013/pdf/ar-threats-2013-508.pdf.
64. Plutarch, *Lives of the Noble Greeks and Romans: Artaxerxes*, http://www.bostonleadershipbuilders.com/plutarch/artaxerxes.htm.
65. Debora Mackenzie, "Renaissance Rulers Plotted Biowar with Hats," *New Scientist*, November 25, 2015, https://www.newscientist.com/article/mg22830494-400-17th-century-plot-to-use-plague-hats-as-bioweapons-revealed/.
66. Michael B. A. Oldstone, *Viruses, Plagues, and History: Past, Present, and Future* (Oxford, UK: Oxford University Press, 2009), p. 64.
67. Judith Miller, "When Germ Warfare Happened," *City Journal*, Spring 2010, http://www.city-journal.org/2010/20_2_germ-warfare.html.
68. John Kelly, *The Great Mortality: An Intimate History of the Black Death, the Most Devastating Plague of All Time* (New York: HarperCollins, 2005), p. 36.
69. Drisdelle, *Parasites.*
70. N. Myhrvold, *Strategic Terrorism: A Call to Action*, Lawfare Research Paper Series 2, 2013.
71. Transcript of Colin Powell's UN Presentation, February 5, 2003, available at https://www.cnn.com/2003/US/02/05/sprj.irq.powell.transcript/index.htm.
72. Myhrvold, *Strategic Terrorism.*
73. Steven Pinker, *Enlightenment Now: The Case for Reason, Science, Humanism, and Progress* (New York: Viking, 2018), p. 307.
74. John Mueller and Mark G. Stewart, *Terror, Security, and Money: Balancing the Risks, Benefits, and Costs of Homeland Security* (Oxford, UK: Oxford University Press, 2011).

Chapter Eleven: Flattening the Plague Cycle

1. Roy Porter, *Disease, Medicine and Society in England, 1550–1860*, vol. 3 (Cambridge, UK: Cambridge University Press, 1995), p. 56.

2. Dorothy Porter, *Health, Civilization and the State: A History of Public Health from Ancient to Modern Times* (Abingdon, UK: Routledge, 2005), p. 122.
3. UNAIDS press release "UNAIDS Report Shows that 19 Million of the 35 Million People Living with HIV Today Do Not Know That They Have the Virus," July 2014, http://www.unaids.org/en/resources/presscentre/pressreleaseandstatement archive/2014/july/20140716prgapreport/.
4. Dean T. Jamison et al. (eds.), *Disease Control Priorities in Developing Countries* (Washington, DC: World Bank Publications, 2006).
5. Dean T. Jamison et al., "Global Health 2035: A World Converging Within a Generation," *Lancet* 382, no. 9908 (2013): 1898–1955.
6. See World Bank Service Delivery Indicators, http://databank.worldbank.org /data/reports.aspx?source=service-delivery-indicators.
7. Randall M. Packard, *A History of Global Health: Interventions into the Lives of Other Peoples* (Baltimore: JHU Press, 2016).
8. Guy Hutton and M. Varughese, *The Costs of Meeting the 2030 Sustainable Development Goal Targets on Drinking Water, Sanitation, and Hygiene*, World Bank Water and Sanitation Department Technical Paper, 2016.
9. Gates Foundation website, "Gates Foundation Reinvent the Toilet Challenge Strategy Overview," https://www.gatesfoundation.org/What-We-Do/Global -Development/Reinvent-the-Toilet-Challenge.
10. Paul Gertler et al., *How Does Health Promotion Work? Evidence from the Dirty Business of Eliminating Open Defecation*, no. w20997, National Bureau of Economic Research, 2015, and Dean Spears and Sneha Lamba, "Effects of Early-Life Exposure to Sanitation on Childhood Cognitive Skills: Evidence from India's Total Sanitation Campaign," *Journal of Human Resources* 51, no. 2 (2015).
11. Jenifer Ehreth, "The Global Value of Vaccination," *Vaccine* 21, no. 7 (2003): 596–600.
12. Ann Nelson, "The Cost of Disease Eradication: Smallpox and Bovine Tuberculosis," *Annals of the New York Academy of Sciences* 894, no. 1 (1999): 83–91.
13. Donald Henderson, "Eradication: Lessons from the Past," MMWR, December 31, 1999, 48: 16–22, http://www.cdc.gov/mmwr/preview/mmwrhtml/su48a6.htm.
14. Kimberly Elliott, *Feeding the Future or Favoring American Farmers* (Washington, DC: Brookings, 2016).
15. Eric Chatelain and Jean-Robert Ioset, "Drug Discovery and Development for Neglected Diseases: the DNDi Model," *Drug Design, Development and Therapy* 5 (2011): 175.
16. Michael B. A. Oldstone, *Viruses, Plagues, and History: Past, Present, and Future* (Oxford, UK: Oxford University Press. 2009), p. 89.
17. Gavi press release, "GAVI Partners Fulfill Promise to Fight Pneumococcal Disease," June 12, 2009, https://www.gavi.org/news/media-room/gavi-partners-fulfill -promise-fight-pneumococcal-disease.
18. Michael Specter, "Mosquitoes and NIMBYism," *New Yorker*, July 11, 2012. Retrieved from https://www.newyorker.com/news/news-desk/mosquitoes-and-nimbyism.
19. CDC press release, "Ebola Outbreak Is Nearing Possible End in Nigeria and Senegal," September 30, 2014, from http://www.cdc.gov/media/releases/2014 /p0930-nigeria-ebola.html.

20. Miles Ott, Shelly F. Shaw, Richard N. Danila, and Ruth Lynfield, "Lessons Learned from the 1918–1919 Influenza Pandemic in Minneapolis and St. Paul, Minnesota," *Public Health Reports* 122, no. 6 (2007): 803–810.
21. Derek Thompson, "What's Behind South Korea's COVID-19 Exceptionalism?" *Atlantic*, May 6, 2020, https://www.theatlantic.com/ideas/archive/2020/05/whats-south-koreas-secret/611215/.
22. Robert Barro, *Non-Pharmaceutical Interventions and Mortality in U.S. Cities During the Great Influenza Pandemic, 1918–1919*, no. w27049, National Bureau of Economic Research, 2020.
23. Ibid.
24. Sheldon J. Watts, *Epidemics and History: Disease, Power and Imperialism* (New Haven: Yale University Press, 1999), p. 200.
25. Jo Nelson Hays, *The Burdens of Disease: Epidemics and Human Response in Western History* (New Brunswick, NJ: Rutgers University Press, 2009), p. 200.
26. The WTO's Sanitary and Phytosanitary Agreement allows signatories to adopt measures to exceed international standards so long as the measures are backed by scientific evidence.
27. Associated Press, "Cheng Satter Emails: UN Health Agency Resisted Declaring Ebola Emergency," AP Newswire, March 20, 2015. Retrieved from http://time.com/3752822/who-ebola-outbreak-emergency/.
28. WHO Statement on the 1st Meeting of the IHR Emergency Committee on the 2014 Ebola Outbreak in West Africa, http://who.int/mediacentre/news/statements/2014/ebola-20140808/en/.
29. Rachel Glennerster, "How Bad Data Fed the Ebola Epidemic," *New York Times*, January 31, 2015, http://www.nytimes.com/2015/01/31/opinion/how-bad-data-fed-the-ebola-epidemic.html.
30. Charles Kenny, "The WHO Isn't Perfect, but It Needs More Money and Power, Not Less," *Technology Review*, April 15, 2020, https://www.technologyreview.com/2020/04/15/999085/who-trump-funding-cut-bad/.
31. Daniel Bressler and Chris Bakerlee, "Designer Bugs," *Vox*, December 6, 2018, https://www.vox.com/future-perfect/2018/12/6/18127430/superbugs-biotech-pathogens-biorisk-pandemic.
32. Patrick Wintour, "US Stays Away as World Leaders Agree Action on Covid-19 Vaccine," *Guardian*, April 24, 2020, https://www.theguardian.com/world/2020/apr/24/us-stays-away-as-world-leaders-agree-action-on-covid-19-vaccine.

Chapter Twelve: Conclusion: Humanity's Greatest Victory

1. David Adam, "Special Report: The Simulations Driving the World's Response to COVID-19," *Nature*, February 20, 2020, https://www.nature.com/articles/d41586-020-01003-6.
2. Victoria Hansen, Eyal Oren, Leslie K. Dennis, and Heidi E. Brown, "Infectious Disease Mortality Trends in the United States, 1980–2014," *JAMA* 316, no. 20 (2016): 2149–2151.

Bibliography

Aberth, John. *The Black Death: The Great Mortality of 1348–1350: A Brief History with Documents*. London: Palgrave Macmillan, 2005.

Adler, Michael W. "The Terrible Peril: A Historical Perspective on the Venereal Diseases," *British Medical Journal* 281, no. 6234 (1980): 206–211.

Aghion, Philippe, Peter Howitt, and Fabrice Murtin. *The Relationship Between Health and Growth: When Lucas Meets Nelson-Phelps*. No. w15813, National Bureau of Economic Research, 2010.

Albanesi, Stefania, and Claudia Olivetti. *Gender Roles and Medical Progress*. No. w14873, National Bureau of Economic Research, 2009.

Allen, Arthur. *The Fantastic Laboratory of Dr. Weigl: How Two Brave Scientists Battled Typhus and Sabotaged the Nazis*. New York: WW Norton & Company, 2009.

Alsan, Marcella. "The Effect of the Tsetse Fly on African Development." *American Economic Review* 105, no. 1 (2015): 382–410.

Alsan, Marcella, and Claudia Goldin. *Watersheds in Infant Mortality: The Role of Effective Water and Sewerage Infrastructure, 1880 to 1915*. No. w21263, National Bureau of Economic Research, 2015.

Amon, Joseph J., and Katherine W. Todrys. "Fear of Foreigners: HIV-Related Restrictions on Entry, Stay, and Residence." *Journal of the International AIDS Society* 11, no. 1 (2008): 8.

Amouzou, Agbessi, et al. "Reduction in Child Mortality in Niger: A Countdown to 2015 Country Case Study." *Lancet* 380, no. 9848 (2012): 1169–1178.

Amulree, Lord. "Hygienic Conditions in Ancient Rome and Modern London," *Medical History* 17, no. 3 (1973): 244–255.

Andersen, Thomas Barnebeck, Peter S. Jensen, and Christian Volmar Skovsgaard. *The Heavy Plough and the Agricultural Revolution in Medieval Europe*. Discussion Papers on Business and Economics, University of Southern Denmark 6, 2013.

Anderson, E. S. "The Problem and Implications of Chloramphenicol Resistance in the Typhoid Bacillus." *Journal of Hygiene* 74, no. 2 (1975): 289–299.

Anderson, Mark, Kerwin Kofi Charles, and Daniel Rees, *Public Health Efforts and the Decline in Urban Mortality*, IZA Discussion Paper No. 11773, 2018.

Angeles, Luis. "Demographic Transitions: Analyzing the Effects of Mortality on Fertility." *Journal of Population Economics* 23, no. 1 (2010): 99–120.

Archibugi, Daniele, and Kim Bizzarri. "The Global Governance of Communicable Diseases: The Case for Vaccine R&D." *Law & Policy* 27, no. 1 (2005): 33–51.

Armstrong, Gregory L., Laura A. Conn, and Robert W. Pinner. "Trends in Infectious Disease Mortality in the United States During the 20th Century." *JAMA* 281, no. 1 (1999): 61–66.

Arora, Suchit. "Health, Human Productivity, and Long-Term Economic Growth." *Journal of Economic History* 61, no. 3 (2001): 699–749.

Asensi-Botet, Francesc. "Fighting Against Smallpox Around the World: The Vaccination Expedition of Xavier de Balmis (1803–1806) and Josep Salvany (1803–1810)." *Contributions to Science* 8, no. 1 (2012): 99–105.

Ashenburg, Katherine. *The Dirt on Clean.* New York: North Point Press, 2007.

Baird, Sarah, et al. *Worms at Work: Long-Run Impacts of Child Health Gains.* Mimeo, University of California at Berkeley, 2011.

Bajardi, Paolo, et al. "Human Mobility Networks, Travel Restrictions, and the Global Spread of 2009 H1N1 Pandemic." *PLoS ONE* 6, no. 1 (2011): e16591.

Banerjee, Abhijit V., and Esther Duflo. "The Economic Lives of the Poor." *Journal of Economic Perspectives* 21, no.1 (2007): 141.

Barnett, Michael L., and Jeffrey A. Linder. "Antibiotic Prescribing to Adults with Sore Throat in the United States, 1997–2010." *JAMA Internal Medicine* 174, no. 1 (2014): 138–140.

Barnosky, Anthony D., and Emily L. Lindsey. "Timing of Quaternary Megafaunal Extinction in South America in Relation to Human Arrival and Climate Change." *Quaternary International* 217, no. 1-2 (2010): 10–29.

Barofsky, Jeremy, et al. *The Economic Effects of Malaria Eradication: Evidence from an Intervention in Uganda.* Program on the Global Demography of Aging Working Paper 70, 2011.

Barreca, Alan I. "The Long-Term Economic Impact of In Utero and Postnatal Exposure to Malaria." *Journal of Human Resources* 45, no. 4 (2010): 865–892.

Barrett, Ronald, et al. "Emerging and Re-Emerging Infectious Diseases: The Third Epidemiologic Transition." *Annual Review of Anthropology* (1988): 247–271.

Barro, Robert. *Non-Pharmaceutical Interventions and Mortality in U.S. Cities During the Great Influenza Pandemic, 1918–1919.* No. w27049, National Bureau of Economic Research, 2020.

Barro, Robert and Jong-Wha Lee. "A New Data Set of Educational Attainment in the World, 1950–2010." *Journal of Development Economics* 104 (2010): 184–198.

Battutah, Ibn, and Tim Mackintosh-Smith. *The Travels of Ibn Battutah.* Pan Macmillan, 2003.

Bazalgette, Joseph William. *On the Main Drainage of London, and the Interception of the Sewage from the River Thames.* London: W. Clowes and Sons, 1865.

Beardsley, Edward H. "Allied Against Sin: American and British Responses to Venereal Disease in World War I." *Medical History* 20, no. 2 (1976): 189–202.

Belfer-Cohen Anna, and Ofer Bar-Yosef. "Early Sedentism in the Near East." In Kuijt, I. (ed.). *Life in Neolithic Farming Communities. Fundamental Issues in Archaeology.* Boston: Springer, 2002.

Benton-Short, Lisa, M. D. Price, and S. Friedman. "Globalization from Below: The Ranking of Global Immigrant Cities. *International Journal of Urban and Regional Research* 29, no. 4 (2005): 945–959.

Bernstein, William. *A Splendid Exchange: How Trade Shaped the World.* New York: Grove/Atlantic, Inc., 2009.

Bhalotra, Sonia et. al. *Urban Water Disinfection and Mortality Decline in Developing Countries.* University of Essex Institute for Social and Economic Research Working Paper 2017-04.

Bhatta, Prakash, P. Simkhada, E. Van Teijlingen, and S. Maybin. "A Questionnaire Study of Voluntary Service Overseas (VSO) Volunteers: Health Risk and Problems Encountered." *Journal of Travel Medicine* 16, no. 5 (2009): 332–337.

Birchenall, Javier. *Disease and Diversity in Africa's Long-Term Economic Development.* Working paper, University of California at Santa Barbara.

Bleakley, Hoyt. "Disease and Development: Evidence from Hookworm Eradication in the American South." *Quarterly Journal of Economics* 122, no. 1 (2007): 73.

Bleakley, Hoyt. "Malaria Eradication in the Americas: A Retrospective Analysis of Childhood Exposure." *American Economic Journal. Applied Economics* 2, no. 2 (2010): 1–45.

Bleakley, Hoyt, and Fabian Lange. "Chronic Disease Burden and the Interaction of Education, Fertility, and Growth." *Review of Economics and Statistics* 91, no. 1 (2009): 52–65.

Bloom, David E., and David Canning. *Global Demographic Change: Dimensions and Economic Significance.* No. w10817. National Bureau of Economic Research, 2004.

Bocquet-Appel, Jean-Pierre. "When the World's Population Took Off: The Springboard of the Neolithic Demographic Transition." *Science* 333, no. 6042 (2011): 560–561.

Boddice, Robert. *Edward Jenner.* Cheltenham, UK: History Press, 2015.

Bollyky, Thomas J. *Plagues and The Paradox of Progress: Why the World Is Getting Healthier in Worrisome Ways.* Cambridge, MA: MIT Press, 2018.

Bos, Kirsten I., et al. "Pre-Columbian Mycobacterial Genomes Reveal Seals as a Source of New World Human Tuberculosis." *Nature* 514 (2014): 494.

Boserup, Ester. *The Conditions of Agricultural Growth: The Economics of Agrarian Change Under Population Pressure.* London: George Allen and Unwin 1965.

Boylston, Arthur. "The Origins of Inoculation." *Journal of the Royal Society of Medicine* 105, no. 7 (2012): 309–313.

Brandt, Allan M. "AIDS in Historical Perspective: Four Lessons from the History of Sexually Transmitted Diseases." *American Journal of Public Health* 78, no. 4 (1988): 367–371.

Bray, R. S. *Armies of Pestilence: The Impact of Disease on History.* Cambridge, UK: James Clarke & Co., 2004.

Burnet, Macfarlane, and David White. *Natural History of Infectious Disease.* 4th ed. Cambridge University Press, 1972.

Burns, Andrew, Dominique Van der Mensbrugghe, and Hans Timmer. *Evaluating the Economic Consequences of Avian Influenza.* Mimeo, World Bank, 2006.

Cantor, Norman F. *In the Wake of the Plague: The Black Death and the World It Made.* New York: Simon & Schuster, 2001.

Carter, W. Hodding. *Flushed: How the Plumber Saved Civilization.* New York: Simon & Schuster, 2007.

Cartwright, Frederick Fox, and Michael Denis Biddiss. *Disease and History*. New York: Marboro Books, 1972.

Cashdan, Elizabeth, and Matthew Steele. "Pathogen Prevalence, Group Bias, and Collectivism in the Standard Cross-Cultural Sample." *Human Nature* 24, no. 1 (2013): 59–75.

Catillon, Maryaline, David Cutler, and Thomas Getzen. *Two Hundred Years of Health and Medical Care: The Importance of Medical Care for Life Expectancy Gains.* No. w25330. National Bureau of Economic Research, 2018.

Cattaneo, Matias D., et al. "Housing, Health, and Happiness." *American Economic Journal: Economic Policy* (2009): 75–105.

Cervellati, Matteo et al. *Malaria Risk and Civil Violence.* Munich Discussion Paper 2017-8. University of Munich, 2017.

Chamberlain, Geoffrey. "British Maternal Mortality in the 19th and Early 20th Centuries." *Journal of the Royal Society of Medicine* 99, no. 11 (2006): 559–563.

Chan, Kam Wing. "The Chinese Hukou System at 50." *Eurasian Geography and Economics* 50, no. 2 (2009): 197–221.

Chang, Ha-Joon. *Economics: The User's Guide*. New York: Bloomsbury Publishing, 2014.

Chatelain, Eric, and Jean-Robert Ioset. "Drug Discovery and Development for Neglected Diseases: The DNDi Model." *Drug Design, Development and Therapy* 5 (2011): 175.

Chavez, Edgar, et al. *Eradicating Polio in Afghanistan and Pakistan.* Mimeo, Center for Strategic and International Studies, 2012.

Clark, Gregory. *A Farewell to Alms: A Brief Economic History of the World.* Princeton, NJ: Princeton University, 2007.

Clement, Charles R., et al. "The Domestication of Amazonia Before European Conquest." *Proceedings of the Royal Society B* 282, no. 1812 (2015).

Cobey, Sarah. "Modeling Infectious Disease Dynamics." *Science* (April 24, 2020).

Cohen, Daniel, and Laura Leker. *Health and Education: Another Look with the Proper Data.* No. 9940. CEPR Discussion Papers.

Cohen, Mark Nathan. *Health and the Rise of Civilization.* New Haven: Yale University Press, 1989.

Colgrove, James. "The McKeown Thesis: A Historical Controversy and Its Enduring Influence." *American Journal of Public Health* 92, no. 5 (2002): 725–729.

Columbus, Christopher. *The Four Voyages of Christopher Columbus*, translated by John Cohen, vol. 217. London: Penguin UK, 1969.

Comas, Iñaki, Mireia Coscolla, Tao Luo, Sonia Borrell, Kathryn E. Holt, Midori Kato-Maeda, Julian Parkhill et al. "Out-of-Africa Migration and Neolithic Coexpansion of Mycobacterium Tuberculosis with Modern Humans." *Nature Genetics* 45, no. 10 (2013): 1176.

Cook, C. Justin. *Long Run Health Effects of the Neolithic Revolution: The Natural Selection of Infectious Disease Resistance.* Mimeo, Yale School of Public Health, 2013.

Cook, Noble David. *Born to Die: Disease and New World Conquest, 1492–1650*, vol. 1. Cambridge, UK: Cambridge University Press, 1998.

Cortes, Hernán. *Letters from Mexico*, translated by Don Pascual de Gayangos. New York: Barnes and Noble, 2012.

Cosgrove, Sara, and Yehuda Carmeli. "The Impact of Antimicrobial Resistance on Health and Economic Outcomes." *Antimicrobial Resistance* 36 (2003): 1433.

Crawford, Dorothy. *Deadly Companions: How Microbes Shaped Our History*. Oxford, UK: Oxford University Press, 2007.

Crawford, Dorothy. *The Invisible Enemy: A Natural History of Viruses*. Oxford University Press, 2000.

Crowley, Roger. *City of Fortune: How Venice Ruled the Seas*. New York: Random House, 2012.

Curtin, Philip, et al. *African History from Earliest Times to Independence*. Pearson, 1995.

Curtin, Philip D. *Death by Migration: Europe's Encounter with the Tropical World in the Nineteenth Century*. Cambridge, UK: Cambridge University Press, 1989.

Curtis, Valerie, et al. "Disgust as an Adaptive System for Disease Avoidance Behavior." *Philosophical Transactions of the Royal Society of London. Series B, Biological Sciences* 366, no. 1563 (2011): 389–401.

Curtis, Valerie, and Sandy Cairncross. "Effect of Washing Hands with Soap on Diarrhoea Risk in the Community: A Systematic Review." *Lancet Infectious Diseases*, no. 3 (2003): 275–281.

Damme, Catherine. "Infanticide: The Worth of an Infant Under Law." *Medical History* 22, no. 1 (1978): 1.

Dargay, Joyce, Dermot Gately, and Martin Sommer. "Vehicle Ownership and Income Growth, Worldwide: 1960–2030." *Energy Journal* (2007): 143–170.

David, Paul A., S. Ryan Johansson, and Andrea Pozzi. *The Demography of an Early Mortality Transition: Life Expectancy, Survival and Mortality Rates for Britain's Royals, 1500–1799*. University of Oxford Discussion Papers in Economic and Social History, no. 83, August 2010.

de Las Cases, Emmanuel. *Mémorial de Sainte-Hélène*. Lecointe, 1828.

Demeure, Christian E., Olivier Dussurget, Guillem Mas Fiol, Anne-Sophie Le Guern, Cyril Savin, and Javier Pizarro-Cerdá. "*Yersinia pestis* and Plague: An Updated View on Evolution, Virulence Determinants, Immune Subversion, Vaccination, and Diagnostics." *Genes & Immunity* 20, no. 5 (2019): 357–370.

Denevan, W. M. "After 1492: Nature Rebounds." *Geographical Review* 106, no. 3 (2016): 381–398.

De Onis, Mercedes, Monika Blössner, and Elaine Borghi. "Global Prevalence and Trends of Overweight and Obesity Among Preschool Children." *American Journal of Clinical Nutrition* 92, no. 5 (2010): 1257–1264.

De Vries, Robert, et al. "Three Mutations Switch H7N9 Influenza to Human-Type Receptor Specificity." *PLoS Pathogens* 13, no. 6 (2017): e1006390.

Dobbs, R., et al. *Urban World: Mapping the Economic Power of Cities*. McKinsey Global Institute, 2011.

Dobson, Andrew P., and E. Robin Carper. "Infectious Diseases and Human Population History." *Bioscience* 46, no. 2 (1996): 115–126.

Drisdelle, Rosemary. *Parasites: Tales of Humanity's Most Unwelcome Guests*. Berkeley: University of California Press, 2010.

Drucker, Ernest, Phillip G. Alcabes, and Preston A. Marx. "The Injection Century: Massive Unsterile Injections and the Emergence of Human Pathogens." *Lancet* 358, no. 9297 (2001): 1989–1992.

Duggan, Ana T., Maria F. Perdomo, Dario Piombino-Mascali, Stephanie Marciniak, Debi Poinar, Matthew V. Emery, Jan P. Buchmann et al. "17th Century Variola Virus Reveals the Recent History of Smallpox." *Current Biology* 26, no. 24 (2016): 3407–3412.

Dunn, Robert R., et al. "Global Drivers of Human Pathogen Richness and Prevalence." *Proceedings of the Royal Society of London B: Biological Sciences* (2010): rspb20100340.

Dupont, B., A. Gandhi, and T. J. Weiss. *The American Invasion of Europe: The Long Term Rise in Overseas Travel, 1820–2000.* No. w13977. National Bureau of Economic Research, 2008.

Easterly, William, and Ross Levine. "Tropics, Germs, and Crops: How Endowments Influence Economic Development." *Journal of Monetary Economics* 50, no. 1 (2003): 3–39.

Echenberg, Myron. "Pestis Redux: The Initial Years of the Third Bubonic Plague Pandemic, 1894–1901." *Journal of World History* 13, no. 2 (2002): 429–449.

Ehreth, Jenifer. "The Global Value of Vaccination." *Vaccine* 21, no. 7 (2003): 596–600.

Elliott, Kimberly. *Feeding the Future or Favoring American Farmers.* Brookings, 2016.

Engerman, Stanley L., and Kenneth L. Sokoloff. *Factor Endowments, Inequality, and Paths of Development Among New World Economics.* No. w9259. National Bureau of Economic Research, 2002.

Esposito, Elena. *Side Effects of Immunities: the African Slave Trade.* Working Paper No. MWP2015/09. European University Institute, 2015.

Evans, Alice, and Liam Swiss. *Why Do Cities Tend to Disrupt Gender Ideologies and Inequalities?* Mimeo, Cambridge University, 2017.

Evans, D. "A Good Riddance of Bad Rubbish? Scatological Musings on Rubbish Disposal and the Handling of 'Filth' in Medieval and Early Post-Medieval Towns." In De Groote, Koen, Dries Tys, and Marnix Pieters (eds.). *Exchanging Medieval Material Culture: Studies on Archaeology and History Presented to Frans Verhaeghe* (2010): 267–278.

Fajgelbaum, P. D., and A. K. Khandelwal. *Measuring the Unequal Gains from Trade.* No. w20331. National Bureau of Economic Research, 2014.

Faria, Nuno R., et al. "The Early Spread and Epidemic Ignition of HIV-1 in Human Populations." *Science* 346, no. 6205 (2014): 56–61.

Farrell, Jeanette. *Invisible Enemies: Stories of Infectious Disease.* New York: Farrar Straus and Giroux, 1998.

Fazal, Tanisha M. "Dead Wrong?: Battle Deaths, Military Medicine, and Exaggerated Reports of War's Demise." *International Security* 39, no. 1 (2014): 95–125.

Feachem, Richard G. A., et al. "Shrinking the Malaria Map: Progress and Prospects." *Lancet* 376, no. 9752 (2010): 1566–1578.

Fenwick, A. "The Global Burden of Neglected Tropical Diseases." *Public Health* 126, no. 3 (2012): 233–236.

Finer, Samuel Edward. *The Life and Times of Sir Edwin Chadwick.* Abingdon-on-Thames: Routledge, 2016.

Fischhoff, B., P. Slovic, S. Lichtenstein, S. Read, and B. Combs. "How Safe Is Safe Enough? A Psychometric Study of Attitudes Towards Technological Risks and Benefits." *Policy Sciences* 9, no. 2 (1978): 127–152

Fogli, Alessandra, and Laura Veldkamp. *Germs, Social Networks and Growth*. No. w18470. National Bureau of Economic Research, 2012.

Fontaine, Olivier, and Charlotte Newton. "A Revolution in the Management of Diarrhoea." *Bulletin of the World Health Organization* 79, no. 5 (2001): 471–472.

Frankenberg, Elizabeth, Jessica Y. Ho, and Duncan Thomas. *Biological Health Risks and Economic Development.* No. w21277. National Bureau of Economic Research, 2015.

Furceri, Davide, Prakash Loungani, Jonathan D. Ostry, and Pietro Pizzuto. "Will Covid-19 Affect Inequality? Evidence from Past Pandemics." *Covid Economics* 12 (2020): 138–157.

Furuse, Yuki, Akira Suzuki, and Hitoshi Oshitani. "Origin of Measles Virus: Divergence from Rinderpest Virus Between the 11th and 12th Centuries." *Virology Journal* 7 (2010): 52.

Galor, Oded. "The Demographic Transition and the Emergence of Sustained Economic Growth." *Journal of the European Economic Association* 3, no. 2-3 (2005): 494–504.

Galor, Oded, and Omer Moav. *The Neolithic Revolution and Contemporary Variations in Life Expectancy.* No. 2007-14. Working Paper, Brown University, Department of Economics, 2007.

Gandhi, Mahatma. *A Guide to Health*. Aukland, NZ: The Floating Press, 2014.

Gat, Azar. *The Causes of War and the Spread of Peace: But Will War Rebound?* Oxford, UK: Oxford University Press, 2017.

Gat, Azar. "Proving Communal Warfare Among Hunter-Gatherers: The Quasi-Rousseauan Error." *Evolutionary Anthropology: Issues, News, and Reviews* 24, no. 3 (2015): 111–126.

Gertler, Paul, et al. *How Does Health Promotion Work? Evidence from the Dirty Business of Eliminating Open Defecation.* No. w20997. National Bureau of Economic Research, 2015.

Geruso, Michael, and Dean Spears. *Sanitation and Health Externalities: Resolving the Muslim Mortality Paradox.* University of Texas at Austin Working Paper, 2014.

Ghodke, Yogita, et al. "HLA and Disease." *European Journal of Epidemiology* 20, no. 6 (2005): 475–488.

Glaeser, Edward, and David Mar. "Cities and Skills," *Journal of Labor Economics* 19, no. 2 (2001): 316–342.

Gómez, José, and Miguel Verdú. "Network Theory May Explain the Vulnerability of Medieval Human Settlements to the Black Death Pandemic." *Nature Scientific Reports* 7 (2017): 43467.

Gráda, Cormac Ó. *Famine: A Short History*. Princeton, NJ: Princeton University Press, 2009.

Grammaticos, Philip C., and Aristidis Diamantis. "Useful Known and Unknown Views of the Father of Modern Medicine, Hippocrates and His Teacher Democritus." *Hellenic Journal of Nuclear Medicine* 11, no. 1 (2008): 2–4.

Grau, L. W., and W. A. Jorgensen. "Medical Support in a Counter-Guerrilla War: Epidemiologic Lessons Learned in the Soviet-Afghan War." *Eye* 2 (1995): 4–58.

Green, Monica. "The Globalisations of Disease." In N. Boivin, R. Crassard, and M. Petraglia (eds.). *Human Dispersal and Species Movement: From Prehistory to the Present.* Cambridge: Cambridge University Press, 2017, pp. 494–520.

Green, Monica. "Taking 'Pandemic' Seriously: Making the Black Death Global." *Medieval Globe* 1, no. 1 (2016).

Guégan, Jean-François, et al. "Disease Diversity and Human Fertility." *Evolution* 55, no. 7 (2001): 1308–1314.

Guernier, Vanina, Michael E. Hochberg, and Jean-François Guégan. "Ecology Drives the Worldwide Distribution of Human Diseases." *PLoS Biology* 2, no. 6 (2004): e141.

Guinnane, Timothy W. "The Historical Fertility Transition: A Guide for Economists." *Journal of Economic Literature* 49, no. 3 (2011): 589–614.

Güneş, Pınar Mine. "The Role of Maternal Education in Child Health: Evidence from a Compulsory Schooling Law." *Economics of Education Review* 47 (2015): 1–16.

Halliday, Stephen. "Death and Miasma in Victorian London: An Obstinate Belief." *British Medical Journal* 323, no. 7327 (2001): 1469.

Hamilton, Marcus J., Robert S. Walker, and Dylan C. Kesler. "Crash and Rebound of Indigenous Populations in Lowland South America." *Scientific Reports* 4 (2014).

Hamusse, Shallo Daba, Taye T. Balcha, and Tefera Belachew. "The Impact of Indoor Residual Spraying on Malaria Incidence in East Shoa Zone, Ethiopia." *Global Health Action* 5 (2012).

Hansen, Casper Worm. *The Effect of Life Expectancy on Schooling: Evidence from the International Health Transition.* Discussion Papers of Business and Economics, University of Southern Denmark, 2012.

Hansen, Victoria, Eyal Oren, Leslie K. Dennis, and Heidi E. Brown. "Infectious Disease Mortality Trends in the United States, 1980–2014." *JAMA* 316, no. 20 (2016): 2149–2151.

Harbeck, M., et al. "*Yersinia pestis* DNA from Skeletal Remains from the 6th Century CE Reveals Insights into Justinianic Plague." *PLoS Pathogens* 9, no. 5 (2013).

Hargarten, Stephen W., and S. P. Baker. "Fatalities in the Peace Corps. A Retrospective Study: 1962 Through 1983." *JAMA* 254 (1985): 1326–1329.

Harkins, Kelly M., and Anne C. Stone. "Ancient Pathogen Genomics: Insights into Timing and Adaptation." *Journal of Human Evolution* 79 (2015): 137–149.

Harper, Kristin N., et al. "On the Origin of the Treponematoses: A Phylogenetic Approach." *PLoS Neglected Tropical Diseases* 2, no. 1 (2008): e148.

Harper, Kyle. *The Fate of Rome: Climate, Disease, and the End of an Empire*. Princeton, NJ: Princeton University Press, 2017.

Harper, Kyle. "Pandemics and Passages to Late Antiquity: Rethinking the Plague of c. 249–270 Described by Cyprian." *Journal of Roman Archaeology* 28 (2015): 223–260.

Harris, Bernard. "Public Health, Nutrition, and the Decline of Mortality: The McKeown Thesis Revisited." *Social History of Medicine* 17, no. 3 (2004): 379–407.

Harrison, Mark. *Disease and the Modern World: 1500 to the Present Day*. New York: John Wiley & Sons, 2013.

Harrison, Mark. "A Global Perspective: Reframing the History of Health, Medicine, and Disease." *Bulletin of the History of Medicine* 89, no. 4 (2015): 639–689.

Hart, Benjamin L. "Behavioral Adaptations to Pathogens and Parasites: Five Strategies." *Neuroscience & Biobehavioral Reviews* 14, no. 3 (1990): 273–294.

Hays, Jo Nelson. *The Burdens of Disease: Epidemics and Human Response in Western History*. New Brunswick, NJ: Rutgers University Press, 2009.

Hendrix, Cullen S., and Kristian Skrede Gleditsch. "Civil War: Is It All About Disease and Xenophobia? A Comment on Letendre, Fincher & Thornhill." *Biological Reviews* 87, no. 1 (2012): 163–167.

Herodotus. *The Histories of Herodotus*. New York: Penguin Books, 1954.

Hilton, Rodney. "The English Rising of 1381." *Marxism Today*, June 17-19, 1981.

Hong, Sok Chul. "The Burden of Early Exposure to Malaria in the United States, 1850–1860: Malnutrition and Immune Disorders." *Journal of Economic History* 67, no. 4 (2007): 1001–1035.

Hopkins, Donald R. *The Greatest Killer: Smallpox in History*. Chicago: University of Chicago Press, 2002.

Huang, Julie Y., Alexandra Sedlovskaya, Joshua M. Ackerman, and John A. Bargh. "Immunizing Against Prejudice: Effects of Disease Protection on Attitudes Toward Out-Groups." *Psychological Science* 22, no. 12 (2011): 1550–1556.

Huigang, Liang, Xiang Xiaowei, Huang Cui, Ma Haixia, and Yuan Zhiming. "A Brief History of the Development of Infectious Disease Prevention, Control, and Biosafety Programs in China."*Journal of Biosafety and Biosecurity* 2, no. 2 (2020).

Human Security Report Project. *Human Security Report* 2009/2010*: The Causes of Peace and the Shrinking Costs of War*. Human Security Report Project, Simon Fraser University, Canada; Oxford University Press, 2011.

Humphries, Jane, and Jacob Weisdorf. "The Wages of Women in England, 1260–1850." *Journal of Economic History* 75, no. 2 (2015): 405–447.

Huskinson, Janet. *Roman Children's Sarcophagi: Their Decoration and Its Social Significance*. Oxford, UK: Oxford University Press, 1996.

Hutton, Guy, and M. Varughese. *The Costs of Meeting the 2030 Sustainable Development Goal Targets on Drinking Water, Sanitation, and Hygiene*. World Bank Water and Sanitation Department Technical Paper, 2016.

Jamison, Dean T., et al. (eds.) *Disease Control Priorities in Developing Countries*. Washington, DC: World Bank Publications, 2006.

Jamison, Dean T., et al. "Global Health 2035: A World Converging Within a Generation." *Lancet* 382, no. 9908 (2013): 1898–1955.

Jannetta, A. B. *Epidemics and Mortality in Early Modern Japan*. Princeton, NJ: Princeton University Press, 2014.

Jannetta, A. "Jennerian Vaccination and the Creation of a National Public Health Agenda in Japan, 1850–1900." *Bulletin of the History of Medicine* (2009): 125–140.

Jayachandran, Seema. *Fertility Decline and Missing Women*. No. w20272. National Bureau of Economic Research, 2014.

Jones, Charles I., and Paul M. Romer "The New Kaldor Facts: Ideas, Institutions, Population, and Human Capital." *American Economic Journal: Macroeconomics* 2, no. 1 (2010): 224–245.

Jones, David S., Scott H. Podolsky, and Jeremy A. Greene. "The Burden of Disease and the Changing Task of Medicine." *New England Journal of Medicine* 366, no. 25 (2012): 2333–2338.

Kalemli-Ozcan, Sebnem. "AIDS Reversal of the Demographic Transition and Economic Development: Evidence from Africa." *Journal of Population Economics* 25, no. 3 (2012): 871–897.

Kaplan, Jed O., et al. "Holocene Carbon Emissions as a Result of Anthropogenic Land Cover Change." *Holocene* 1 (2010): 17.

Kaplan, Jed O., Kristen M. Krumhardt, and Niklaus Zimmermann. "The Prehistoric and Preindustrial Deforestation of Europe." *Quaternary Science Reviews* 28, no. 27 (2009): 3016–3034.

Karlsson, Elinor K., Dominic P. Kwiatkowski, and Pardis C. Sabeti. "Natural Selection and Infectious Disease in Human Populations." *Nature Reviews Genetics* 15, no. 6 (2014): 379.

Karwowski, Maciej, Marta Kowal, Agata Groyecka, Michał Białek, Izabela Lebuda, Agnieszka Sorokowska, and Piotr Sorokowski. *When in Danger, Turn Right: Covid-19 Threat Promotes Social Conservatism and Right-Wing Presidential Candidates.* Mimeo, University of Wrocław, 2020.

Katona, Peter, and Judit Katona-Apte. "The Interaction Between Nutrition and Infection." *Clinical Infectious Diseases* 46, no.10 (2008): 1582–1588.

Kazanjian, Powel. "Ebola in Antiquity?" *Clinical Infectious Diseases* 61, no. 6 (2015): 963–968.

Kelly, John. *The Great Mortality: An Intimate History of the Black Death, the Most Devastating Plague of All Time.* New York: HarperCollins Publishers, 2005.

Kemper, Alex, Matthew Davis, and Gary Freed. "Expected Adverse Events in a Mass Smallpox Vaccination Campaign." *Effective Clinical Practice* 5 (2002): 84–90.

Kenny, Charles. *Getting Better: Why Global Development Is Succeeding—and How We Can Improve the World Even More.* New York: Basic Books, 2012.

Kenny, Charles. *The Upside of Down: Why the Rise of the Rest Is Good for the West.* New York: Basic Books, 2014.

Kenny, Charles, and Dev Patel. *Norms and Reform: Legalizing Homosexuality Improves Attitudes.* CGD Working Paper 465. Washington, DC: Center for Global Development, 2017.

Kerwin, Jason T. *The Effect of HIV Infection Risk Beliefs on Risky Sexual Behavior: Scared Straight or Scared to Death?* Job Market Paper, University of Michigan, 2014.

Khan, Fahd, et al. "The Story of the Condom." *Indian Journal of Urology, IJU: Journal of the Urological Society of India* 29, no. 1 (2013): 12.

Klein, Herbert S. "The First Americans: The Current Debate." *Journal of Interdisciplinary History* 46, no. 4 (2016): 543–562.

Klein Goldewijk, Kees, et al. "The HYDE 3.1 Spatially Explicit Database of Human-Induced Global Land-Use Change over the Past 12,000 Years." *Global Ecology and Biogeography* 20, no. 1 (2011): 73–86.

Koch, A., C. Brierley, M. M. Maslin, and S. L. Lewis. "Earth System Impacts of the European Arrival and Great Dying in the Americas After 1492." *Quaternary Science Reviews* 207 (2019): 13–36.

Korpela, Katri, et al. "Intestinal Microbiome Is Related to Lifetime Antibiotic Use in Finnish Pre-School Children." *Nature Communications* 7 (2016).

Kraut, Alan M. "Foreign Bodies: The Perennial Negotiation over Health and Culture in a Nation of Immigrants." *Journal of American Ethnic History* (2004): 3–22.

La Porta, Rafael, Florencio Lopez-de-Silanes, and Andrei Shleifer. "The Economic Consequences of Legal Origins." *Journal of Economic Literature* 46, no. 2 (2008): 285–332.

Larson, H. J., et al. "The State of Vaccine Confidence 2016: Global Insights Through a 67-Country Survey." *EBioMedicine* 12 (2016): 295–301.

Latham, Ronald. Introduction to *Marco Polo: The Travels*. New York: Penguin, 1958.

Lawson, Nicholas, and Dean Spears. *What Doesn't Kill You Makes You Poorer: Adult Wages and the Early-Life Disease Environment in India.* World Bank Policy Research Working Paper 7121, 2014.

Lefèber, Yvonne, and Henk W. A. Voorhoeve. *Indigenous Customs in Childbirth and Child Care*. Assen, Netherlands: Uitgeverij Van Gorcum, 1998.

Letendre, Kenneth, Corey L. Fincher, and Randy Thornhill. "Does Infectious Disease Cause Global Variation in the Frequency of Intrastate Armed Conflict and Civil War?" *Biological Reviews* 85, no. 3 (2010): 669–683.

Leung, Angela Ki Che. "Organized Medicine in Ming-Qing China: State and Private Medical Institutions in the Lower Yangzi Region." *Late Imperial China* 8, no. 1 (1987): 134–166.

Lewis, Simon L., and Mark A. Maslin. "Defining the Anthropocene." *Nature* 519, no. 7542 (2015): 171–180.

Little, Lester K. "Life and Afterlife of the First Plague Pandemic." In Little, Lesster K. (ed.). *Plague and the End of Antiquity* (2007): 1.

Liu, Jenny, et al. "Malaria Eradication: Is It Possible? Is It Worth It? Should We Do It?" *Lancet Global Health* 1, no. 1 (2013): e2–e3.

Livi-Bacci, Massimo. *A Concise History of World Population.* New York: John Wiley and Sons, 2012.

Llamas, Bastien, Lars Fehren-Schmitz, Guido Valverde, Julien Soubrier, Swapan Mallick, Nadin Rohland, Susanne Nordenfelt, et al. "Ancient Mitochondrial DNA Provides High-Resolution Time Scale of the Peopling of the Americas." *Science Advances* 2, no. 4 (2016).

Lourenço-de-Oliveira, R., et al. "*Aedes aegypti* in Brazil: Genetically Differentiated Populations with High Susceptibility to Dengue and Yellow Fever Viruses." *Transactions of the Royal Society of Tropical Medicine and Hygiene* 98, no. 1 (2004): 43–54.

Lozano, Rafael, et al. "Global and Regional Mortality from 235 Causes of Death for 20 Age Groups in 1990 and 2010: A Systematic Analysis for the Global Burden of Disease Study 2010." *Lancet* 380, no. 9859 (2013): 2095–2128.

Lynch, Susan V., et al. "Effects of Early-Life Exposure to Allergens and Bacteria on Recurrent Wheeze and Atopy in Urban Children." *Journal of Allergy and Clinical Immunology* 134, no. 3 (2014): 593–601.

Macoris, Maria de Lourdes G., et al. "Resistance of *Aedes aegypti* from the State of São Paulo, Brazil, to Organophosphates Insecticides." *Memórias do Instituto Oswaldo Cruz* 98, no. 5 (2003): 703–708.

Maddison, Angus. "The West and the Rest in the World Economy: 1000-2030." *World Economics* 9, no. 4 (2008): 75–99.

Maddison, Angus. *The World Economy Volume 1: A Millennial Perspective, Volume 2: Historical Statistics*. Haryana, India: Academic Foundation, 2007.

Malešević, Siniša. "How Old Is Human Brutality? On the Structural Origins of Violence." *Common Knowledge* 22, no. 1 (2016): 81–104.

Malthus, Thomas Robert. *An Essay on the Principle of Population; or a View of Its Past and Present Effects on Human Happiness, an Inquiry into Our Prospects Respecting the Future Removal or Mitigation of the Evils Which It Occasions.* Edited with an introduction and notes by Geoffrey Gilbert. Oxford, UK: Oxford University Press, 2008.

Mann, Charles C. *1491: New Revelations of the Americas Before Columbus*. New York: Alfred A. Knopf, 2005.

Manring, M. M., et al. "Treatment of War Wounds: A Historical Review." *Clinical Orthopaedics and Related Research* 467, no. 8 (2009): 2168–2191.

Manson, Patrick. "The Malaria Parasite." *Journal of the Royal African Society* 6, no. 23 (1907): 225–233.

Markel, Howard, and Alexandra Minna Stern. "The Foreignness of Germs: The Persistent Association of Immigrants and Disease in American Society." *Milbank Quarterly* 80, no. 4 (2002): 757–788.

McGuire, Robert A., and Philip Coelho. *Parasites, Pathogens, and Progress*. Cambridge, MA: MIT Press, 2011.

McKinlay, John B., and Sonja M. McKinlay. "The Questionable Contribution of Medical Measures to the Decline of Mortality in the United States in the Twentieth Century." *Milbank Memorial Fund Quarterly: Health and Society* (1977): 405–428.

McLaughlin, Raoul. *Rome and the Distant East: Trade Routes to the Ancient Lands of Arabia, India and China*. London: Bloomsbury Publishing, 2010.

McNeill, William. *Plagues and Peoples*. New York: Anchor, 1996.

Michalopoulos, Stelios, and Elias Papaioannou. "Further Evidence on the Link Between Pre-Colonial Political Centralization and Comparative Economic Development in Africa." *Economics Letters* 126 (2015): 57–62.

Montag, Josef. *Legal Origins and Labor Market Outcomes of Men and Women.* SSRN Working Paper Series, 2011.

Morelli, Giovanna, Yajun Song, Camila J. Mazzoni, Mark Eppinger, Philippe Roumagnac, David M. Wagner, Mirjam Feldkamp, et al. "*Yersinia pestis* Genome Sequencing Identifies Patterns of Global Phylogenetic Diversity." *Nature Genetics* 42, no. 12 (2010): 1140–1143.

Morens, David M., Gregory K. Folkers, and Anthony S. Fauci. "The Challenge of Emerging and Re-Emerging Infectious Diseases." *Nature* 430, no. 6996 (2004): 242–249.

Morens, David M., Gregory K. Folkers, and Anthony S. Fauci. "Emerging Infections: A Perpetual Challenge." *Lancet Infectious Diseases* 8, no. 11 (2008): 710–719.

Mortensen, Chad R., et al. "Infection Breeds Reticence: The Effects of Disease Salience on Self-Perceptions of Personality and Behavioral Avoidance Tendencies." *Psychological Science* 21 (2010): 440–447.

Mueller, John, and Mark G. Stewart. *Terror, Security, and Money: Balancing the Risks, Benefits, and Costs of Homeland Security*. Oxford, UK: Oxford University Press, 2011.

Müller, Miriam. "Conflict and Revolt: The Bishop of Ely and His Peasants at the Manor of Brandon in Suffolk c. 1300–81." *Rural History* 23, no. 1 (2012): 1–19.

Mulligan, Casey B. *Economic Activity and the Value of Medical Innovation During a Pandemic.* University of Chicago Becker Friedman Institute for Economics Working Paper 2020-48.

Murray, Damian R., Russell Trudeau, and Mark Schaller. "On the Origins of Cultural Differences in Conformity: Four Tests of the Pathogen Prevalence Hypothesis." *Personality and Social Psychology Bulletin* 37, no. 3 (2011): 318–329.

Myhrvold N. *Strategic Terrorism : A Call to Action.* The Lawfare Research Paper Series 2, 2013.

Nagaoka, L., T. Rick, and S. Wolverton. "The Overkill Model and Its Impact on Environmental Research." *Ecology and Evolution* 8, no. 19 (2018): 9683–9696.

Naraya, D., et al. *Voices of the Poor: Can Anyone Hear Us?* (English). New York: Oxford University Press, 2000.

Nayyar, Gaurvika M. L., et al. "Poor-Quality Antimalarial Drugs in Southeast Asia and Sub-Saharan Africa." *Lancet Infectious Diseases* 12, no. 6 (2012): 488–496.

Nelson, Ann. "The Cost of Disease Eradication: Smallpox and Bovine Tuberculosis." *Annals of the New York Academy of Sciences* 894, no. 1 (1999): 83–91.

Nickell, Zachary D., and Matthew D. Moran. "Disease Introduction by Aboriginal Humans in North America and the Pleistocene Extinction." *Journal of Ecological Anthropology* 19, no.1 (2017): 2.

Nowrasteh, Alex, and Andrew Forrester. *How US Travel Restrictions on China Affected the Spread of Covid-19 in the United States.* Cato Working Paper no. 58, 2020.

Nugent, Rachel, Emma Back, and Alexandra Beith. *The Race Against Drug Resistance.* Washington, DC: Center for Global Development, 2010.

Nunn, Nathan. "The Long-Term Effects of Africa's Slave Trades." *Quarterly Journal of Economics* 1, no. 23 (2008): 139–176.

Nunn, Nathan, and Leonard Wantchekon. "The Slave Trade and the Origins of Mistrust in Africa." *American Economic Review* 101 (2011): 3221–3252.

Nunn, Nathan, and Nancy Qian. "The Columbian Exchange: A History of Disease, Food, and Ideas." *Journal of Economic Perspectives* 24, no. 2 (2010): 63–188.

Nutton, Vivian. "The Seeds of Disease: An Explanation of Contagion and Infection from the Greeks to the Renaissance." *Medical History* 27, no. 1 (1983): 1–34.

Obikili, Nonso. *The Trans-Atlantic Slave Trade and Local Political Fragmentation in Africa.* Economic Research South Africa Working Paper 406, 2014.

Offit, Paul A. *Vaccinated: One Man's Quest to Defeat the World's Deadliest Diseases.* Washington, DC: Smithsonian Books, 2007.

Oldstone, Michael B. A. *Viruses, Plagues, and History: Past, Present and Future.* Oxford, UK: Oxford University Press, 1998.

Oster, Emily. "HIV and Sexual Behavior Change: Why Not Africa?" *Journal of Health Economics* 31, no. 1 (2012): 35–49.

Oster, Emily. "Routes of Infection: Exports and HIV Incidence in Sub-Saharan Africa." *Journal of the European Economic Association* 10, no. 5 (2012): 1025–1058.

Oster, Emily, Ira Shoulson, and E. Dorsey. "Limited Life Expectancy, Human Capital and Health Investments." *American Economic Review* 103, no. 5 (2013): 1977–2002.

Ott, Miles, Shelly F. Shaw, Richard N. Danila, and Ruth Lynfield. "Lessons Learned from the 1918–1919 Influenza Pandemic in Minneapolis and St. Paul, Minnesota." *Public Health Reports* 122, no. 6 (2007): 803–810.

Packard, Randall M. *A History of Global Health: Interventions into the Lives of Other Peoples*. Baltimore: JHU Press, 2016.

Palloni, Alberto, and Randy Wyrick. "Mortality Decline in Latin America: Changes in the Structure of Causes of Deaths, 1950–1975." *Social Biology* 28, no. 3-4 (1981): 187–216.

Pamuk, Şevket. "The Black Death and the Origins of the 'Great Divergence' Across Europe, 1300–1600." *European Review of Economic History* 11, no. 3 (2007): 289–317.

Papagrigorakis, M. J., et al. "DNA Examination of Ancient Dental Pulp Incriminates Typhoid Fever as a Probable Cause of the Plague of Athens." *International Journal of Infectious Diseases* 10, no. 3 (2006): 206–214.

Pennington, R. "Hunter-Gatherer Demography." In Panter-Brick, C., R. H. Layton, and P. Rowley-Conwy (eds.). *Hunter-Gatherers: An Interdisciplinary Perspective* (Cambridge: Cambridge University Press, 2001).

Pepin, Jacques, et al. "Evolution of the Global Burden of Viral Infections from Unsafe Medical Injections, 2000–2010." *PloS One* 9, no. 6 (2014).

Percoco, Marco. *The Fight Against Geography: Malaria and Economic Development in Italian Regions*. FEEM Working Paper 07, 2011.

Persson, Sheryl. *Smallpox, Syphilis and Salvation: Medical Breakthroughs That Changed the World*. Dunedin, NZ: Exisle Publishing, 2010.

Peters, Margaret. *Labor Markets After the Black Death: Landlord Collusion and the Imposition of Serfdom in Eastern Europe and the Middle East*. Mimeo, prepared for the Stanford Comparative Politics Workshop, 2010.

Phadke, Varun, et al. "Association Between Vaccine Refusal and Vaccine-Preventable Diseases in the United States: A Review of Measles and Pertussis." *JAMA* 315, no. 11 (2016): 1149–1158.

Piel, Frédéric B., et al. "Global Distribution of the Sickle Cell Gene and Geographical Confirmation of the Malaria Hypothesis." *Nature Communications* 1 (2010): 104.

Pinker, Steven. *The Better Angels of Our Nature: Why Violence Has Declined*. New York: Penguin Books, 2012.

Pinker, Steven. *Enlightenment Now: The Case for Reason, Science, Humanism, and Progress*. New York: Viking, 2018.

Polo, Marco. *The Travels*, translated by Ronald Latham. New York: Penguin, 1958.

Porter, Dorothy. *Health, Civilization and the State: A History of Public Health from Ancient to Modern Times*. Abingdon, UK: Routledge, 1999.

Porter, Dorothy, and Roy Porter. "The Politics of Prevention: Anti-Vaccinationism and Public Health in Nineteenth-Century England." *Medical History* 32, no. 3 (1988): 231–252.

Porter, Roy. *Disease, Medicine and Society in England, 1550–1860*, vol. 3. Cambridge University Press, 1995.

President's Council of Advisors on Science and Technology (PCAST). *Combating Antibiotic Resistance*. Washington, DC: The White House, 2014.

Putterman, Louis, and David N. Weil. *Post-1500 Population Flows and the Long Run Determinants of Economic Growth and Inequality*. No. w14448. National Bureau of Economic Research, 2008.

Raoult, Didier, et al. "Evidence for Louse-Transmitted Diseases in Soldiers of Napoleon's Grand Army in Vilnius." *Journal of Infectious Diseases* 193, no. 1 (2006): 112–120.

Rascovan, Nicolás, Karl-Göran Sjögren, Kristian Kristiansen, Rasmus Nielsen, Eske Willerslev, Christelle Desnues, and Simon Rasmussen. "Emergence and Spread of Basal Lineages of Yersinia Pestis During the Neolithic Decline." *Cell* 176, no. 1-2 (2019): 295–305.

Rassy, Dunia, and Richard D. Smith. "The Economic Impact of H1N1 on Mexico's Tourist and Pork Sectors." *Health Economics* 22, no. 7 (2013): 824–834.

Rees Clayton, E. M., M. Todd, J. B. Dowd, and A. E. Aiello. "The Impact of Bisphenol A and Triclosan on Immune Parameters in the U.S. Population, NHANES 2003–2006." *Environmental Health Perspectives* 119, no. 3 (2011): 390–396.

Ridley, Matt. *The Red Queen: Sex and the Evolution of Human Nature.* London: Penguin UK, 1994.

Riley, James C. *Rising Life Expectancy: A Global History*. Cambridge, UK: Cambridge University Press, 2001.

Rosen, William. *Justinian's Flea: Plague, Empire and the Birth of Europe*. New York: Random House, 2010.

Rothschild, Bruce M., et al. "First European Exposure to Syphilis: The Dominican Republic at the Time of Columbian Contact." *Clinical Infectious Diseases* 31, no. 4 (2000): 936–941.

Ruddiman, William F. "How Did Humans First Alter Global Climate?" *Scientific American* 292, no. 3 (2005): 46–53.

Sachs, Jeffrey, and Pia Malaney. "The Economic and Social Burden of Malaria." *Nature* 415, no. 6872 (2002): 680–685.

Saito, Osamu. "Forest History and the Great Divergence." *Journal of Global History* 4, no. 3 (2009): 379–404.

Sallares, Robert, Abigail Bouwman, and Cecilia Anderung. "The Spread of Malaria to Southern Europe in Antiquity: New Approaches to Old Problems." *Medical History* 48, no. 3 (2004): 311–328.

Sanche, S., Y. T. Lin, C. Xu, E. Romero-Severson, N. Hengartner, and R. Ke. "High Contagiousness and Rapid Spread of Respiratory Syndrome Coronavirus 2." *Emerging Infectious Diseases* 26, no. 7 (2020).

Schaller, Mark, and Damian Murray. "Infectious Disease and the Creation of Culture." *Advances in Culture and Psychology* 1 (2011): 99–151.

Scheidel, Walter. "Emperors, Aristocrats, and the Grim Reaper: Towards a Demographic Profile of the Roman Elite." *Classical Quarterly* 49, no. 1 (1999): 254–281.

Scott, James C. *Against the Grain: A Deep History of the First Civilizations*. New Haven: Yale University Press, 2017.

Serwadda, David, et al. "Slim Disease: A New Disease in Uganda and Its Association with HTLV-III Infection." *Lancet* 326, no. 8460 (1985): 849–852.

Sherman, Paul W., and Jennifer Billing. "Darwinian Gastronomy: Why We Use Spices." *BioScience* 49, no. 6 (1999): 453–463.

Shrestha, Sundar S., et al. "Estimating the Burden of 2009 Pandemic Influenza A (H1N1) in the United States (April 2009–April 2010)." *Clinical Infectious Diseases* 52, suppl. 1 (2011): S75–S82.

Silverman, Sarah Kelly. *The 1363 English Sumptuary Law: A Comparison with Fabric Prices of the Late Fourteenth-Century.* Thesis Presented in Partial Fulfillment of the Requirements for the Degree Master of Science in the Graduate School of the Ohio State University by Graduate Program in Human Ecology. The Ohio State University, 2011.

Smith, Katherine F., et al. "Global Rise in Infectious Disease Outbreaks." *Journal of the Royal Society Interface* 11 (2014): 20140950.

Soares, Rodrigo R. "On the Determinants of Mortality Reductions in the Developing World." *Population and Development Review* 33, no. 2 (2007): 247–287.

Spears, Dean, and Sneha Lamba. "Effects of Early-Life Exposure to Sanitation on Childhood Cognitive Skills: Evidence from India's Total Sanitation Campaign." *Journal of Human Resources* 51, no. 2 (2015).

Spielman, Andrew, and Michael d'Antonio. *Mosquito: The Story of Man's Deadliest Foe.* New York: Hyperion, 2002.

Stearns, Peter N. *Childhood in World History.* Abingdon-on-Thames, UK: Routledge, 2005.

Steckel, Richard H. *The Best of Times, the Worst of Times: Health and Nutrition in Pre-Columbian America.* No. w10299. National Bureau of Economic Research, 2004.

Steckel, Richard H., and Joseph M. Prince. "Tallest in the World: Native Americans of the Great Plains in the Nineteenth Century." *American Economic Review* 91, no. 1 (2001): 287.

SteelFisher, Gillian K., Robert J. Blendon, and Narayani Lasala-Blanco. "Ebola in the United States—Public Reactions and Implications." *New England Journal of Medicine* 373, no. 9 (2015): 789–791.

Steinberg, J. "AIDS Prevention Is Thicker Than Blood. Zimbabwe." *Links* 9, no. 2 (1991): 3.

Sussman, G. D. "Was the Black Death in India and China?" *Bulletin of the History of Medicine* (2011): 319–355.

Suzuki, Akihito. "Smallpox and the Epidemiological Heritage of Modern Japan: Towards a Total History." *Medical History* 55, no. 3 (2011): 313–318.

Szreter, Simon. "The Importance of Social Intervention in Britain's Mortality Decline c. 1850–1914: A Re-interpretation of the Role of Public Health." *Social History of Medicine* 1, no. 1 (1988): 1–38.

Tacoli, Cecilia, Gordon McGranahan, and David Satterthwaite. "Urbanization, Poverty and Inequity: Is Rural-Urban Migration a Poverty Problem or Part of the Solution." *New Global Frontier: Urbanization, Poverty and Environment in the 21st Century* (2008): 37–53.

Talty, Stephan. *The Illustrious Dead: The Terrifying Story of How Typhus Killed Napoleon's Greatest Army.* New York: Crown Publishers, 2009.

Tasca, Cecilia, et al. "Women and Hysteria in the History of Mental Health." *Clinical Practice & Epidemiology in Mental Health* 8, no. 1 (2012).

Tatem, Andrew J., David J. Rogers, and S. I. Hay. "Global Transport Networks and Infectious Disease Spread." *Advances in Parasitology* 62 (2006): 293–343.

Teso, Edoardo. *The Long-Term Effect of Demographic Shocks on the Evolution of Gender Roles: Evidence from the Trans-Atlantic Slave Trade.* Mimeo, Harvard University, 2016.

Thibaudeau, Antoine-Claire. *Bonaparte and the Consulate*. New York: The Macmillan Company, 1908.

Thomas, Hugh. *Conquest: Montezuma, Cortes and the Fall of Old Mexico.* New York: Simon & Schuster, 1994.

Thucydides. *The History of the Peloponnesian War*, translated by David Grene. Chicago: University of Chicago Press, 1989, pp. 115–118.

Tilman, David, et al. "Agricultural Sustainability and Intensive Production Practices." *Nature* 418, no. 6898 (2002): 671–677.

Todd, Jim, et al. "Editorial: Measuring HIV-Related Mortality in the First Decade of Anti-Retroviral Therapy in Sub-Saharan Africa." *Global Health Action* 7 (May 2014).

Tognotti, Eugenia. "Lessons from the History of Quarantine, from Plague to Influenza A." *Emerging Infectious Diseases* 19, no. 2 (2013): 254.

Togoobaatar, Ganchimeg, et al. "Survey of Non-Prescribed Use of Antibiotics for Children in an Urban Community in Mongolia." *Bulletin of the World Health Organization* 88, no. 12 (2010): 930–936.

Tomes, Nancy. "The Making of a Germ Panic, Then and Now." *American Journal of Public Health* 90, no. 2 (2000): 191.

Toynbee, Arnold. *A Study of History.* Abridgement of vols. I–VI by D. C. Somervell. New York: Oxford University Press, 1974.

Trambaiolo, D. "Vaccination and the Politics of Medical Knowledge in Nineteenth-Century Japan." *Bulletin of the History of Medicine* 88, no. 3 (2014): 431-456.

Trape, Jean-François, et al. "Malaria Morbidity and Pyrethroid Resistance After the Introduction of Insecticide-Treated Bednets and Artemisinin-Based Combination Therapies: A Longitudinal Study." *Lancet Infectious Diseases* 11, no. 12 (2011): 925–932.

Tybur, Joshua M., et al. "Extending the Behavioral Immune System to Political Psychology: Are Political Conservatism and Disgust Sensitivity Really Related?" *Evolutionary Psychology* 8, no. 4 (2010): 147470491000800406.

Valdiserri, Ron O. "*Cum hastis sic clypeatis:* The Turbulent History of the Condom." *Bulletin of the New York Academy of Medicine* 64, no. 3 (1988): 237.

van Leeuwen, Florian, et al. "Regional Variation in Pathogen Prevalence Predicts Endorsement of Group-Focused Moral Concerns." *Evolution and Human Behavior* 33, no. 5 (2012): 429–437.

van Panhuis, Willem G., et al. "Contagious Diseases in the United States from 1888 to the Present." *New England Journal of Medicine* 369, no. 22 (2013): 2152.

Voigtländer, Nico, and Hans-Joachim Voth. *How the West "Invented" Fertility Restriction.* No. w17314. National Bureau of Economic Research, 2011.

Voigtländer, Nico, and Hans-Joachim Voth. "Persecution Perpetuated: The Medieval Origins of Anti-Semitic Violence in Nazi Germany." *Quarterly Journal of Economics* 127, no. 3 (2012a): 1339–1392.

Voigtländer, Nico, and Hans-Joachim Voth. "The Three Horsemen of Riches: Plague, War, and Urbanization in Early Modern Europe." *Review of Economic Studies* (2012b): rds034.

Voth, Hans-Joachim. "Living Standards and the Urban Environment." *Cambridge Economic History of Modern Britain* 1 (2004): 1700–1860.

Walter, Jakob. *Diary of a Napoleonic Foot Soldier*. New York: Doubleday, 2012.

Wang, Shiyon, P. Marquez, and John Langenbrunner. "Toward a Healthy and Harmonious Life in China: Stemming the Rising Tide of Non-Communicable Diseases." Mimeo. The World Bank, 2011.

Watts, Sheldon J. *Epidemics And History: Disease, Power and Imperialism*. New Haven: Yale University Press, 1999.

Wertheim, J. O., M. D. Smith, D. M. Smith, K. Scheffler, and S. L. Kosakovsky Pond. "Evolutionary Origins of Human Herpes Simplex Viruses 1 and 2." *Molecular Biology and Evolution* 31, no. 9 (2014): 2356–2364.

Wheelis, Mark. "Biological Warfare at the 1346 Siege of Caffa." *Emerging Infectious Diseases* 8, no. 9 (2002): 971–975.

Wilkins, Ernest H. "Petrarch's Coronation Oration." *Publications of the Modern Language Association of America* (1953): 1241–1250.

Witt, Ronald. "Francesco Petrarca and the Parameters of Historical Research." *Religions* 3, no. 3 (2012): 699–709.

Wolfe, Nathan D., Claire Panosian Dunavan, and Jared Diamond. "Origins of Major Human Infectious Diseases." *Nature* 447, no. 7142 (2007): 279–283.

Woods, Robert. "Mortality in Eighteenth-Century London: A New Look at the Bills." *Local Population Studies* 77 (2006): 12.

Wootton, David. *Bad Medicine: Doctors Doing Harm Since Hippocrates*. Oxford, UK: Oxford University Press, 2007.

World Health Organization. *The World Medicines Situation*. World Health Organization, 2004.

World Health Organization. *World Health Statistics 2012*. World Health Organization, 2012.

Wrigley, Edward. *People, Cities and Wealth: The Transformation of Traditional Society*. Oxford, UK: Oxford University Press, 1987.

Wrigley, Edward Anthony. *Poverty, Progress, and Population*. Cambridge, UK: Cambridge University Press, 2004.

Yap, Mui Teng. "Fertility and Population Policy: The Singapore Experience." *Journal of Population and Social Security (Population)* 1 (2003): 643–658.

Younger, Stephen D. *Cross-Country Determinants of Declines in Infant Mortality: A Growth Regression Approach*. Cornell Food and Nutrition Policy Program Working Paper 130, 2001.

Zinsser, Hans. *Rats, Lice and History*. Piscataway, NJ: Transaction Publishers, 2007.

Index

Page numbers in *italics* refer to illustrations.